P9-CCM-560

Patient Safety

Guest Editor

JUAN A. SANCHEZ, MD, MPA, FACS

SURGICAL CLINICS
OF NORTH AMERICA

www.surgical.theclinics.com

Consulting Editor
RONALD F. MARTIN, MD

February 2012 • Volume 92 • Number 1

SAUNDERS an imprint of ELSEVIER, Inc.

W.B. SAUNDERS COMPANY
A Division of Elsevier Inc.
1600 John F. Kennedy Blvd., Suite 1800, Philadelphia, PA 19103-2899
http://www.surgical.theclinics.com
SURGICAL CLINICS OF NORTH AMERICA Volume 92, Number 1
February 2012 ISSN 0039–6109, ISBN-13: 978-1-4557-3937-0
Editor: John Vassallo, j.vassallo@elsevier.com
Developmental Editor: Teia Stone

Surgical Clinics of North America (ISSN 0039–6109) is published bimonthly by Elsevier Inc., 360 Park Avenue South, New York, NY 10010-1710. Months of publication are February, April, June, August, October, and December. Business and Editorial Offices: 1600 John F. Kennedy Blvd., Suite 1800, Philadelphia, PA 19103-2899. Periodicals postage paid at New York, NY and additional mailing offices. Subscription prices are $339.00 per year for US individuals, $575.00 per year for US institutions, $166.00 per year for US students and residents, $415.00 per year for Canadian individuals, $714.00 per year for Canadian institutions, $468.00 for international individuals, $714.00 per year for international institutions and $229.00 per year for Canadian and foreign students/residents. To receive student/resident rate, orders must be accompanied by name of affiliated institution, date of term, and the *signature* of program/residency coordinator on institution letterhead. Orders will be billed at individual rate until proof of status is received. Foreign air speed delivery is included in all *Clinics* subscription prices. All prices are subject to change without notice. POSTMASTER: Send address changes to *Surgical Clinics*, Elsevier Health Sciences Division, Subscription Customer Service, 3251 Riverport Lane, Maryland Heights, MO 63043. **Customer Service (orders, claims, online, change of address): Telephone: 1-800-654-2452 (U.S. and Canada); 314-447-8871 (outside U.S. and Canada). Fax: 314-447-8029. E-mail: journalscustomerservice-usa@elsevier.com (for print support); journalsonline support-usa@elsevier.com (for online support).**

Reprints. For copies of 100 or more, of articles in this publication, please contact the Commercial Reprints Department, Elsevier Inc., 360 Park Avenue South, New York, New York 10010-1710. Tel. (212) 633-3812, Fax: (212) 462-1935, e-mail: reprints@elsevier.com.

The Surgical Clinics of North America is also published in Spanish by McGraw-Hill Interamericana Editores S.A., P.O. Box 5-237 06500 Mexico D.F. Mexico; and in Portuguese by Interlivros Edicoes Ltda., Rua Comandante Coelho 1085, CEP 21250, Rio de Janeiro, Brazil; and in Greek by Paschalidis Medical Publications, Athens Greece.

The Surgical Clinics of North America is covered in *MEDLINE/PubMed (Index Medicus), EMBASE/Excerpta Medica, Current Contents/Clinical Medicine, Current Contents/Life Sciences, Science Citation Index,* and *ISI/BIOMED.*

Printed in the United States of America.

Contributors

CONSULTING EDITOR

RONALD F. MARTIN, MD
Staff Surgeon, Department of Surgery, Marshfield Clinic, Marshfield, Wisconsin; Clinical Associate Professor, University of Wisconsin School of Medicine and Public Health, Madison, Wisconsin; Colonel, Medical Corps, United States Army Reserve

GUEST EDITOR

JUAN A. SANCHEZ, MD, MPA, FACS
Chairman and Program Director, Department of Surgery, Saint Mary's Hospital, Waterbury; Professor of Surgery, University of Connecticut Health Center, Farmington, Connecticut

AUTHORS

PAUL R. BARACH, MD, MPH
Visiting Professor, Utrecht Medical Centre, University of Utrecht, Utrecht, Netherlands; University of Stavanger, School of Nursing and Midwifery, Stavanger, Norway

BRYCE R. CASSIN, RN, BA (Hons), AFCHSM
Lecturer, University of Western Sydney, School of Nursing and Midwifery; PhD Candidate, University of Technology, School of the Built Environment, Sydney, New South Wales, Australia

MICHOL COOPER, MD, PhD
Department of Surgery, Johns Hopkins Hospital, Baltimore, Maryland

EDWARD J. DUNN, MD, ScD
Adjunct Professor of Health Policy and Management, University of Kentucky College of Public Health, Louisville; Chief of Performance Improvement and an Ethics Consultant, Lexington VA Medical Center, Louisville, Kentucky

AALIYAH EAVES-LEANOS, JD, PhD
Health Law Attorney, Bioethicist and Former National Center for Patient Safety Fellow (2009–2010), Risk Manager and Ethics Consultant, Lexington VA Medical Center, Lexington, Kentucky

ANDREW W. ELBARDISSI, MD, MPH
Clinical Fellow in Surgery, Division of Cardiac Surgery, Brigham and Women's Hospital; Department of Surgery, Brigham and Women's Hospital and the Center for Surgery and Public Health, Harvard Medical School, Boston, Massachusetts

iv   Contributors

SCOTT J. ELLNER, DO, MPH, FACS
Director of Surgical Quality, Department of Surgery, Saint Francis Hospital and Medical Center, Hartford, Connecticut; Assistant Professor of Surgery, University of Connecticut Medical School, Farmington, Connecticut

JACOB GALLINGER, BA
The Wilson Centre for Research in Medical Education, University Health Network and University of Toronto, Toronto, Ontario, Canada

PAUL W. JOYNER, MD
Chief Surgical Resident, University of Connecticut Residency Program in General Surgery, Department of Surgery, University of Connecticut Health Center, Farmington, Connecticut

MARY CATHERINE KARL, MBA
Principal, Surgical Safety Institute, Tampa, Florida

RICHARD KARL, MD, FACS
Chairman Emeritus, Department of Surgery, University of South Florida; Founder, Surgical Safety Institute, Tampa, Florida

KEVIN W. LOBDELL, MD
Director of Quality and Program Director, Cardiothoracic Surgery, Sanger Heart and Vascular Institute, Carolinas HealthCare System; Clinical Professor of Surgery, University of North Carolina, School of Medicine, Charlotte, North Carolina

SHELLY LUU, BSc
The Wilson Centre for Research in Medical Education, University Health Network and University of Toronto; Faculty of Medicine, University of Toronto, Toronto, Ontario, Canada

MARTIN A. MAKARY, MD, MPH
Department of Surgery, Johns Hopkins Hospital, Baltimore, Maryland

CAROL-ANNE MOULTON, MBBS, MEd, PhD, FRACS
The Wilson Centre for Research in Medical Education, University Health Network and University of Toronto; Department of Surgery, University of Toronto, Toronto, Ontario, Canada

RUSSELL J. NAUTA, MD, FACS
Professor of Surgery, Chair, Department of Surgery, Harvard Medical School, Mount Auburn Hospital, Cambridge, Massachusetts

SHUK ON ANNIE LEUNG, BASc
The Wilson Centre for Research in Medical Education, University Health Network and University of Toronto; Faculty of Medicine, University of Toronto, Toronto, Ontario, Canada

PRIYANKA PATEL, BSc
The Wilson Centre for Research in Medical Education, University Health Network and University of Toronto; Institute of Medical Science, University of Toronto, Toronto, Ontario, Canada

SIMON PATERSON-BROWN, MBBS, MPhil, MS, FRCS(Edin), FRCS(Engl), FCS(HK)
Consultant General and Upper Gastro-intestinal Surgeon, Honorary Senior Lecturer,
Royal Infirmary of Edinburgh, Edinburgh University, Edinburgh, Scotland,
United Kingdom

JUAN A. SANCHEZ, MD, MPA, FACS
Chairman and Program Director in Surgery, Department of Surgery, Saint Mary's
Hospital, Waterbury; Professor of Surgery, University of Connecticut Health Center,
Farmington, Connecticut

HEENA P. SANTRY, MD, MS
Assistant Professor of Surgery, and Quantitative Health Sciences, Department of Surgery,
University of Massachusetts Medical School, Worcester, Massachusetts

HARRY C. SAX, MD, MHCM
Professor and Vice Chair, Department of Surgery; Senior Physician Liaison, Cedars-Sinai
Medicine Clinical Transformation Initiative, Cedars-Sinai Medical Center, Los Angeles,
California

LAURENT ST-MARTIN, BSc
The Wilson Centre for Research in Medical Education, University Health Network
and University of Toronto; Institute of Medical Science, University of Toronto, Toronto,
Ontario, Canada

SOTIRIS STAMOU, MD, PhD
Assistant Professor of Cardiothoracic Surgery, Fred and Lena Meijer Heart Center,
Michigan State University, Grand Rapids, Michigan

THORALF M. SUNDT, MD
Professor of Surgery, Division of Cardiac Surgery, Massachusetts General Hospital,
Harvard Medical School, Boston, Massachusetts

SHERRY M. WREN, MD
Professor of Surgery, Associate Dean for Academic Affairs, Stanford University School
of Medicine, Stanford, California; Chief of General Surgery, Department of Surgery,
Palo Alto Veterans Hospital, Stanford University Medical School, Palo Alto, California

STEVEN YULE, MA, MSc, PhD, CPsychol
Lecturer in Surgery, Harvard Medical School, Boston; Director of Research and
Education, STRATUS Center for Medical Simulation, Brigham & Women's Hospital,
Boston, Massachusetts; Lecturer in Psychology (Hon.), University of Aberdeen, Scotland,
United Kingdom

Contents

Foreword: Patient Safety   xiii

Ronald F. Martin

Preface: Patient Safety   xvii

Juan A. Sanchez

**High Reliability Organizations and Surgical Microsystems: Re-engineering
Surgical Care**   1

Juan A. Sanchez and Paul R. Barach

> Error prevention and mitigation is the primary goal in high-risk health care, particularly in areas such as surgery. There is growing consensus that significant improvement is hard to come by as a result of the vast complexity and inefficient processes of the health care system. Recommendations and innovations that focus on individual processes do not address the larger and often intangible systemic and cultural factors that create vulnerabilities throughout the entire system. This article introduces basic concepts of complexity and systems theory that are useful in redesigning the surgical work environment to create safety, quality, and reliability in surgical care.

Building High-Performance Teams in the Operating Room   15

Harry C. Sax

> Building effective teams requires the delineation of clear goals, an understanding of each member's role in reaching that goal, and continuous feedback as issues are identified. The solo mentality required to become a health care provider needs to be modified to see a bigger picture. Finally, consistent buy-in and support from senior administration to deal with disruptive personalities is vital for long-term success.

Human Factors and Operating Room Safety   21

Andrew W. ElBardissi and Thoralf M. Sundt

> A human factors model is used to highlight the nature of many systems factors that affect surgical performance, including the OR environment, teamwork and communication, technology and equipment, tasks and workload factors, and organizational variables. If further improvements in the success rate and reliability of cardiac surgery are to be realized, interventions need to be developed to reduce the negative impact that work system failures can have on surgical performance. Some recommendations are proposed here; however, several challenges remain.

Surgeons' Non-technical Skills   37

Steven Yule and Simon Paterson-Brown

> The importance of non-technical skills to surgical performance is gaining wide acceptance. This article discusses the core cognitive and social skills

categories thought to underpin medical knowledge and surgical expertise, and describes the rise of non-technical skill models of assessment in surgery. Behavior rating systems such as NOTSS (Non-Technical Skills for Surgeons) have been developed to support education and assessment in this regard. We now understand more about these critical skills and how they impact surgery. The challenge in the future is to incorporate them into undergraduate teaching, postgraduate training, workplace assessment, and perhaps even selection.

A Comprehensive Unit-Based Safety Program (CUSP) in Surgery: Improving Quality Through Transparency   **51**

Michol Cooper and Martin A. Makary

Many medical errors can be attributed to large and complex health care systems in which care is increasingly fragmented. Hospitals with good safety cultures have lower complication rates, and improved patient and staff satisfaction. Transparency in health care is an increasingly recognized means to improve outcomes by allowing the free market to reward hospitals with a strong safety culture, good outcomes, and compliance with evidence-based medicine. As more data become available regarding strategies that work to improve patient safety and such strategies are more widely implemented, significant improvements in the quality of care that is delivered nationwide should become apparent.

Hospital-Acquired Infections   **65**

Kevin W. Lobdell, Sotiris Stamou, and Juan A. Sanchez

Health-acquired infection (HAI) is defined as a localized or systemic condition resulting from an adverse reaction to the presence of infectious agents or its toxins. This article focuses on HAIs that are well studied, common, and costly (direct, indirect, and intangible). The HAIs reviewed are catheter-related bloodstream infection, ventilator-associated pneumonia, surgical site infection, and catheter-associated urinary tract infection. This article excludes discussion of *Clostridium difficile* infections and vancomycin-resistant *Enterococcus*.

Information Technologies and Patient Safety   **79**

Scott J. Ellner and Paul W. Joyner

Advances in health information technology provide significant opportunities for improvements in surgical patient safety. The adoption and use of electronic health records can enhance communication along the surgical spectrum of care. Bar coding and radiofrequency identification technology are strategies to prevent retained surgical sponges and for tracking the operating room supply chain. Computerized intraoperative monitoring systems can improve the performance of the operating room team. Automated data registries collect patient information to be analyzed and used for surgical quality improvement.

Adverse Events: Root Causes and Latent Factors   **89**

Richard Karl

This article describes the process of root cause analysis (RCA), the theories of error that underlie the concept of systemic or latent factors that allow errors to occur or to be propagated without correction; the difference between the process in health care and those found in high-reliability organizations; and suggests some ways to augment the standard health care RCA into a more robust and helpful process.

Making Sense of Root Cause Analysis Investigations of Surgery-Related Adverse Events   101

Bryce R. Cassin and Paul R. Barach

This article discusses the limitations of root cause analysis (RCA) for surgical adverse events. Making sense of adverse events involves an appreciation of the unique features in a problematic situation, which resist generalization to other contexts. The top priority of adverse event investigations must be to inform the design of systems that help clinicians to adapt and respond effectively in real time to undesirable combinations of design, performance, and circumstance. RCAs can create opportunities in the clinical workplace for clinicians to reflect on local barriers and identify enablers of safe and reliable outcomes.

Residency Training Oversight(s) in Surgery: The History and Legacy of the Accreditation Council for Graduate Medical Education Reforms   117

Russell J. Nauta

Despite a quarter century of discourse since a sentinel event in New York City raised the question of appropriate oversight for graduate medical education, many questions remain unanswered. Even with the Accreditation Council for Graduate Medical Education rules in place, some opportunity remains to examine handoff methodology, the relationship of duty hours to education, and the impact of fatigue on resident performance. Neurophysiologic adjuncts applied concomitantly to evaluation of didactic performance offer promise for data-driven definition of the optimal shift. Concurrently, the merits of specialty-specific oversight of graduate medical education remain under active consideration.

Teaching the Slowing-down Moments of Operative Judgment   125

Laurent St-Martin, Priyanka Patel, Jacob Gallinger, and Carol-anne Moulton

Surgical judgment has been an elusive construct to define, let alone teach or assess. A recent study has characterized a phenomenon called slowing down when you should, and suggests it is a hallmark for operative judgment. This research highlights areas where surgical judgment can be identified and therefore taught more explicitly in the operating room. Through the identification of these slowing-down moments and an understanding of how control is negotiated between surgeon and trainee during these moments, this article uses several theoretic frameworks to understand how teaching judgment in the operating room can be optimized.

The Role of Unconscious Bias in Surgical Safety and Outcomes   137

Heena P. Santry and Sherry M. Wren

Racial, ethnic, and gender disparities in health outcomes are a major challenge for the US health care system. Although the causes of these disparities are multifactorial, unconscious bias on the part of health care providers plays a role. Unconscious bias occurs when subconscious prejudicial beliefs about stereotypical individual attributes result in an automatic and unconscious reaction and/or behavior based on those beliefs. This article reviews the evidence in support of unconscious bias and resultant disparate health outcomes. Although unconscious bias cannot be entirely eliminated, acknowledging it, encouraging empathy, and understanding patients' sociocultural context promotes just, equitable, and compassionate care to all patients.

When Bad Things Happen to Good Surgeons: Reactions to Adverse Events   153

Shelly Luu, Shuk On Annie Leung, and Carol-anne Moulton

Adverse events are, unfortunately, common components of surgical practice. Much has been done to develop safer systems to prevent these adverse events; however, there has been less focus on the surgeon experiencing these events. This article presents a framework to understand surgeons' reactions to adverse events that was derived from a more recent study as well as a review of relevant psychology literatures. This framework is then situated within the broader picture of mindful practice to explore how the psychological and social dimensions of the surgeon can affect judgment and cognition.

Open Disclosure of Adverse Events: Transparency and Safety in Health Care   163

Aaliyah Eaves-Leanos and Edward J. Dunn

Many patients suffering adverse events in health care turn to the legal system to learn what happened to them and to seek compensation. Health care providers have ethical, professional, and legal duties to disclose the harmful effects of care to the patient, regardless of how small the risk. The purpose of open disclosure is to explain what happened to the patient and to seek a just outcome for patient and provider. This article explores our experience of managing and implementing an open disclosure program in an acute and chronic tertiary care facility with university affiliation in the Veterans Health Administration.

Index   179

FORTHCOMING ISSUES

April 2012
Management of Peri-operative Complications
Lewis J. Kaplan, MD, and
Stanley H. Rosenbaum, MD,
Guest Editors

June 2012
Pediatric Surgery
Kenneth S. Azarow, MD, and
Robert A. Cusick, MD,
Guest Editors

August 2012
Recent Advances and Future Directions in Trauma Care
Jeremy Cannon, MD, *Guest Editor*

October 2012
Management of Esophageal Neoplasms
Chadrick E. Denlinger, MD and
Carolyn E. Reed, MD,
Guest Editors

RECENT ISSUES

December 2011
Bariatric and Metabolic Surgery
Shanu N. Kothari, MD, FACS,
Guest Editor

October 2011
Gastric Surgery
George M. Fuhrman, MD,
Guest Editor

August 2011
Nutrition and Metabolism of The Surgical Patient, Part II
Stanley J. Dudrick, MD, and
Juan A. Sanchez, MD,
Guest Editors

June 2011
Nutrition and Metabolism of The Surgical Patient, Part I
Stanley J. Dudrick, MD, and
Juan A. Sanchez, MD, *Guest Editors*

ISSUE OF RELATED INTEREST

Medical Clinics of North America March 2008 (Vol. 92, Issue 2)
Hospital Medicine
Scott A. Flanders, MD, Vikas I. Parekh, MD, and Lakshmi Halasyamani, MD,
Guest Editors

THE CLINICS ARE NOW AVAILABLE ONLINE!

Access your subscription at:
www.theclinics.com

Foreword

Patient Safety

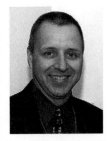

Ronald F. Martin, MD
Consulting Editor

In the United States Army we have an expression—*Everyone* is a safety officer. That expression may exist in the other branches as well but I can only vouch for the Army. At first glance one might think it is one of those catchy slogans that gets tossed about to make everybody feel included. And while it may achieve that to some degree, it also means more. It means that it is not just everyone's opportunity to point out dangerous behavior, but it is also everyone's duty to point out dangerous behavior. The most junior recruit can inform a four-star general that he or she is doing something dangerous and, in theory, it should be well received.

The aviation community has a similar concept in the Crew Resource Management training and practice. A review of some of the more spectacular aviation catastrophes revealed that there was a cultural issue in the aviation community that led to an unnecessary increase for risk under some conditions. Multiple partners in the assessment of safety in the aviation industry, such as the Federal Aviation Administration, National Transportation Safety Board, various pilots and crew organizations, groups such as Flight Safety International, and others have worked collaboratively to make air travel safer for you and me. To the credit of these organizations, they have made a systematic study of failure and have been open with the results. I cannot say that the system is perfect since I do not directly participate in it—perhaps those who do may be able to point out some issues that escape an outsider's perspective—but conceptually it is one of the models worth studying.

We physicians, and particularly we surgeons, have tried to borrow tools and procedures from our aviation brethren for years. My first exposure was at a Surgical Grand Rounds presented by Flight Safety International organized by Dr David Clark of Maine Medical Center during my residency over two decades ago. Dr Clark was always intellectually far ahead of the curve and this was just one more example of that. During the Grand Rounds it became abundantly clear from reviewing the flight data and cockpit voice recordings just how much preventable error existed—and this in an industry

Surg Clin N Am 92 (2012) xiii–xv
doi:10.1016/j.suc.2011.12.007
0039-6109/12/$ – see front matter **surgical.theclinics.com**

where the pilots themselves suffer first on impact! If they were not motivated to improve their system, who would be?

Since that first introduction to this concept I have had the privilege of listening to many presentations on similar topics and how they impact safety. Some have been more focused on procedures and checklists, some on communication styles, some on information transfers, some on fatigue and other topics. They have varied a bit in quality and utility. Some have been thinly veiled attempts to shift control over something (the distinct minority) and some have been so painfully obvious that one has to wonder how it is possible that it wasn't known or studied decades or centuries ago. Independent of the above, they have all still contributed positively to the discussion.

Perhaps with a nod to the aviation industry, we in surgery have pursued simulated environment training on both the individual scale and the team/facility scale (a while ago we dedicated an entire issue of the *Surgical Clinics of North America Clinics* to just that topic) in the hope that would help us improve our outcomes and safety. No matter how hard one tries though, one serious disconnect from aviation safety and patient safety remains: humans designed and built airplanes and while one might cleverly make the argument that humans build humans, we certainly didn't design them. I would submit that there is far less variability among Boeing 737s than there is among even a closely related group of humans, which makes it more challenging to simulate in a meaningful way.

The other major stumbling block in direct comparison of the two industries has to do with the necessity of use of the product or perhaps put into our jargon—indications. When one flies, it is almost always a matter of some choice (at least in commercial or general aviation) and delaying or eliminating the trip altogether usually represents more inconvenience than threat to life. When someone arrives at the hospital in extremis, far more often than not engagement in medical care is not optional nor is it time insensitive. The concept of minimum requirements for providing medical care is far less stringent than for flight. The converse also holds true to a certain degree. There are many procedures or operations that are either elective or debatable as to their overall utility yet they carry many of the same risks as less elective procedures.

I would like to challenge our surgical community a bit if I may. If we were truly serious about improving patient safety, we would approach this topic from several markedly different but ultimately absolutely related approaches. First, we would accept that without a near totality of data acquisition and analysis we are unlikely to recognize real trends and make certain kinds of changes. We require a degree of standardization of data acquisition and reporting from all venues and we should engage seriously in how we analyze the data and distribute the results.

The obvious barriers to this are money, more money, ego, and personal and institutional risk. To be clearer, first it takes money to collect the data and then more money to analyze the data. Those costs must be borne initially but it may be that over time, savings may recoup some or all of those expenses. Ego, well, ego is ego and we have to separate that or we'll never put patients first. Last, every person and every institution would prefer not to have their data made public unless they already know that they are advantaged by the publication of said data. Even if the "competitive" nature of making data available were resolved, there is still the fear of legal reprisal that will always cloud the integrity of voluntarily submitted or self-reported data. If we (society) were really interested in self-preservation through superior medicine, then we would address tort reform to remove this barrier to honest information.

We doctors, though, must make a trade if we want tort reform; we have to allow or engage in better policing of our ranks. Shocking though true—not everybody currently working in the care of the citizenry is good enough to remain on the job. Some may be remediable but others need to move on. We cannot expect the public to call off the lawyers without offering them certain protections in return. Fair is fair.

When it comes to safety, in many respects, it is about the money. I know people say it isn't but it is. In this respect the aviation industry and we suffer along the same lines. For the most part, neither of us gets paid not to work. Also similarly, in aviation one doesn't have to make the trip safer if no one flight occurs and we don't have to improve on the outcomes of operations not performed. Of course, there are differences; very few arrive at the airport wondering if perhaps they need to board a flight. Air travelers are far more aware of their need for flight and the alternatives available to them than the average patient. As long as doctors get paid more to deliver more care independent of quality and timing than to deliver optimal amounts of care in optimal ways, we will most likely slow our progression to better care and increased value to the patient and society.

While we may not be quite there at this instant, we are rapidly approaching a time in which we have the technical capacity to capture and analyze the amount of data needed to understand better our system of patient care. I wish I were as hopeful that we had the societal will to make the changes required or the professional courage to do what is necessary about policing ourselves and investing a bit more of our capital into the broader initiatives of patient safety—but I am not quite ready to hold my breath on either of those at the moment.

In some respects it would almost seem redundant to put out an issue of the *Surgical Clinics of North America* on patient safety. After all, is not everything we study somehow dedicated to the safety of our patients? Yet, taking a step back and looking at not just how can we make better-informed clinical decisions but what can we learn on the industrial side of what we do is necessary. To improve patient safety truly we will have to improve our health care system—yes, it is just as easy as that. Sarcasm put aside, however, who better to drive this than us? Surgeons have always risen to great challenges and we have no reason to abandon that trait now. As always, making great strides requires understanding the topics at hand. Dr Sanchez and his colleagues have provided a series of articles that should inform you and stimulate some to learn more. It is far easier for those of us who are well versed in surgery to learn industry strategies and tactics for safety than it is for industry folk to learn surgery. Promise.

This is one area where we can all make a difference. There is room for improvement on every scale at every facility. As we are taught in the Army, everyone is a safety officer. Perhaps, the world of medicine and the world of surgery would benefit a bit from adopting the same philosophy.

Ronald F. Martin, MD
Department of Surgery
Marshfield Clinic
1000 North Oak Avenue
Marshfield, WI 54449, USA

E-mail address:
martin.ronald@marshfield.org

Preface

Patient Safety

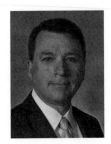

Juan A. Sanchez, MD, MPA
Guest Editor

Perhaps ironically, the tragic sinking of the *RMS Titanic*, most likely as a result of human error, occurred at about same the time that Harvard physician, biochemist, and historian, Lawrence J. Henderson, famously proclaimed that the pace of progress in medicine had reached a point at which a random patient had a better than even chance of benefiting from consultation with a random physician. Since then, the availability of treatment options for virtually every ailment known to afflict humanity has exploded, resulting in an unprecedented growth in the quantity of health care services. These advances, punctuated occasionally by spectacular cures, have delivered a level of societal welfare and productivity that could not have been envisioned by those who first learned of that great nautical catastrophe 100 years ago.

It is becoming increasingly unclear, however, whether this extensive repertoire of available treatments, for all its sophistication and expense, effectively and reliably produces the intended goals of restoring health, alleviating suffering, and prolonging life for all. Moreover, the increased division of labor among members of the health care team has resulted in progressive subspecialization of medical disciplines and in new categories of providers to deliver these services. The unintended consequences created by this level of complexity, including problems with coordination and information exchange, produce measurable deficits in the quality of care and disparities in its distribution. Coupled with these concerns is the increasing realization that payment for all available services, even if optimally deployed and effective, is unsustainable. More importantly, perhaps, questions have surfaced, based on credible and persuasive data, as to whether the care provided can actually be harmful.

While the relatively young patient safety movement and the sciences supporting it continue to develop a theoretical framework and an imperative for change, progress in the actual reduction in preventable adverse events remains slow. Diffusion of knowledge generated by safety research into clinical practice has been difficult. At best, the reaction of many health care organizations, already beleaguered by regulation and oversight, to initiatives such as the Surgical Care Improvement Project, reflect

Surg Clin N Am 92 (2012) xvii–xix
doi:10.1016/j.suc.2011.12.006
0039-6109/12/$ – see front matter © 2012 Elsevier Inc. All rights reserved.

surgical.theclinics.com

a "teaching to the test" mentality without a deeper appreciation of the problems inherent in the increasingly complex socio-technical system we call health care. Thorny, intractable issues of organizational and culture change, based on differing mental models held by various stakeholders, result in cognitive dissonance and passive, if not outright active, resistance.

Those of us on the front lines of surgery are particularly sensitive to issues of error, whether of omission or commission, given our historical and high level of selfless commitment to our patients and to the most exacting standards of performance. As such, any insinuation that we contribute to preventable harm may be difficult to accept but evidence is mounting that some patients are worse off than would be expected after exposure to the health care system. Furthermore, the increasing complexity of the delivery system and the expanding disease burden in society requires us to rethink how we deliver care in a more reliable, evidence-based, and patient-centered manner. The traditional surgical focus on technical precision, dexterity, and patient-level risk assessment will need to be complemented by an expanded appreciation for system-level risk assessment, group dynamics, and other social skills, which, ultimately, also contribute to patient outcomes. Experience in other technically oriented industries has found initial resistance to change when it involves transitioning toward a different paradigm, especially one that involves "soft" skills. In the aviation industry, for example, pilots were known to mock early attempts by the industry at enhancing communication skills by refusing to be sent to "charm school." Now, a climate of safety is embedded throughout the entire industry from suppliers to the control tower. It is not inconceivable, then, that surgery can enjoy similar level of reliability and culture of safety in the near future.

In many ways, these are heady times for those interested in reengineering the delivery of care, particularly surgical care, to maximize effectiveness and reliability. The surgical environment is "target rich" for mitigating hazards. Opportunities for improvement abound. However, meaningful change will require a transition to a more team-oriented, system-based *modus operandi* as well as a deeper awareness of how complex adaptive systems behave. The sciences of human factors, organizational psychology, management science, and those other affiliated disciplines which have transformed other safety-critical industries into ultrasafe and highly reliable endeavors, appear to have increasing relevance to the world of surgery. These perspectives from the social sciences and engineering appear to offer a new lens through which transformative change can occur in health care. This can only happen, however, if individuals inside the surgical "space" embrace these ideas enthusiastically and develop innovative ways to deliver high-quality, safe surgical care.

This volume of *Surgical Clinics of North America* hopes to showcase newer concepts and stimulating ideas related to patient safety that are of relevance to surgeons and others who are involved with the care of surgical patients. While not an exhaustive treatise on safety and human error, the scope of subjects illustrates the multidimensional and interdisciplinary nature of patient safety as applied science. It is anticipated that the reader will come away with a more nuanced understanding of the current adaptive challenges facing surgical "systems" today and will respond to the call to action that is intended to be the subtext of this work.

I am grateful to Dr Ronald F. Martin, Consulting Editor, for the enthusiasm, support, and expansive wisdom of considering patient safety a suitable topic for the *Surgical Clinics of North America* as well as for having the confidence in me to bring together these outstanding experts. Additionally, I would like to thank Mr John Vassallo, Associate Publisher, and the many dedicated people at Elsevier for their commitment to publishing consistently high-quality material. Finally, I would like to express my gratitude to all the contributing authors who, under considerable time constraints, produced content that is clear, coherent, and abundantly provocative. It is my ultimate hope that each reader will feel compelled to consider how their surgical environments can be refocused on safety, reliability, and improved effectiveness.

Juan A. Sanchez, MD, MPA
Department of Surgery
Saint Mary's Hospital
56 Franklin Street
Waterbury, CT 06706, USA
University of Connecticut Health Center
Farmington, CT, USA

E-mail address:
Juan.Sanchez@stmh.org

High Reliability Organizations and Surgical Microsystems: Re-engineering Surgical Care

Juan A. Sanchez, MD, MPA[a,b,]*, Paul R. Barach, MD, MPH[c]

KEYWORDS

- High reliability • Clinical microsystems • Teams • Patient safety
- Safe culture • Normal accident theory

I would not give a fig for the simplicity this side of complexity, but I would give my life for the simplicity on the other side of complexity.
—*Oliver Wendell Holmes Jr[1]*

THE HIGH RELIABILITY ORGANIZATION

The surgical space, by its nature, is a high-risk environment where hazards lurk around every corner and for every patient. The patients who come to surgery are generally among the sickest and at more advanced stages of disease. The very act of treatment involves interventions that are often considerably invasive with vigorous and unpredictable physiologic responses. The level of complexity, both in task-oriented and cognitive demands, results in a dynamic, unforgiving environment that can magnify the consequences of even small lapses and errors.

Other complex sociotechnical systems, which operate in similar environments, have been able to redesign their operations such that they consistently perform at high levels of safety with reliable outcomes. These high reliability organizations (HROs) have characteristics that parallel many features of the surgical environment, including the use of complex technologies, a fast-paced tempo of operations, and a high level of risk, yet they manifest spectacularly low error rates. HROs are required to respond to a wide variety of situations under changing environmental conditions in a reliable and

[a] Department of Surgery, Saint Mary's Hospital, 56 Franklin Street, Waterbury, CT 06706, USA
[b] University of Connecticut Health Center, 263 Farmington Avenue, Farmington, CT 06030, USA
[c] Utrecht Medical Centre, Utrech, The Netherlands
* Corresponding author. Department of Surgery, Saint Mary's Hospital, 56 Franklin Street, Waterbury, CT 06706.
E-mail address: Juan.Sanchez@STMH.ORG

Surg Clin N Am 92 (2012) 1–14
doi:10.1016/j.suc.2011.12.005
0039-6109/12/$ – see front matter © 2012 Elsevier Inc. All rights reserved.

consistent way. Examples of HROs include aircraft carriers, nuclear power plants, and firefighting teams. Weick and Sutcliffe have studied these industries and found that they share an extraordinary capacity to discover and manage unexpected events resulting in exceptional safety and consistent levels of performance despite a fast-changing external environment.[2]

Resilience, Brittleness, and the Law of Stretched Systems

A challenge to HROs is the tendency to stretch systems to their capacity as they continuously strive to improve overall performance. It is the objective of an outstanding management team to enhance efficiency such that throughput is maximized for a given level of input. When financial outcomes are also under consideration, there is a corresponding downward pressure to minimize costs and, therefore, to limit resources and still achieve the desired outcomes in volume and quality. This Law of Stretched Systems, a property of complex and dynamic environments, occurs when exceptionally consistent improvement in performance is required and managed through human decision making without accounting for the possibility of errors and unanticipated variability.[3] This principle posits that every system is ultimately stretched to operate at its capacity as efficiency improves. Innovations such as new information technologies, and performance gains are exploited to achieve a new intensity, complexity of work, and tempo of activity. This coadaptive dynamic results in escalating pressure to do more, faster, and in more complex ways.[4] Health care delivery systems are thought to routinely function at the limits of their capacity. Managers and administrators tend to increase throughput up to efficiency maxima only to be thwarted by unanticipated operational constraints. Surgeons and anesthesiologists are all too familiar with the common bed crunch occurring each morning and the potential for delaying or even canceling scheduled operations.

The ability of a team to activate a repertoire of actions and resources not normally used during standard operations to allow the work to continue through unexpectedly high demand or a failure can build resiliency into a system. This *margin of maneuver,* a concept that resonates with pilots and others in high-hazard environments, provides a cushion for an organization to recover toward normal operational levels. When all ICU beds are occupied in a hospital with a level I trauma program, for example, the system has little or no margin to accept a new major trauma patient. The organization is said to be solid, a condition that reflects its *brittleness*, a manifestation of a stretched system.

The ideas supporting the concept of HROs are germane to the surgical environment. The pace of operations, expectations of superior levels of performance and safety, and the degree of uncertainty in surgery require a systems-based approach. Additionally, high-hazard, safety-critical organizations can reach levels of complexity that result in failure due to data overload, hitting a wall of complexity. The concept of *resilience*, a term borrowed from materials engineering, refers to the properties of a system that allow it to absorb unusual amounts of stress without causing a failure, or a crack, in the integral function of the organization.[5] Two major themes emerge from the examination of HROs.[6] The first theme is anticipation, a state of mindfulness throughout the entire organization in which continuous vigilance for potential sources of harm is expected and practiced as a shared value. This state of mind focuses on preparedness for any and all process failures, surveillance for formal and informal signals, and planning contingencies. The second idea is containment and refers to those actions to be taken immediately when a system fails to advert or mitigate further damage and injury.

HROs Share 5 Key Principles

Preoccupation with failure

HROs treat each event, lapse, or near miss (NM) as a symptom of a system flaw that can have severe consequences, particularly when separate, seemingly insignificant events or violations coincide and produce a catastrophic failure. This is consistent with the human errors framework proposed by James Reason and his Swiss cheese model of accident causation.[7] This preoccupation with failure is coupled with the understanding that small violations and errors are not part of normal process variation and can conspire to cause patient harm.[8] It is difficult, for example, to view a break in the sterile field or a lack of closed loop communication during an operation as a major adverse event in the context of a complex surgical procedure. Yet these unsafe acts can contribute to a catastrophic outcome when combined with other violations and errors until a tipping point is reached. It is easy, alternatively, to develop complacency and a false sense of security when the incidence of patient harm is rare and thus continue to allow deviant behavior to go unchecked.[9] The high reliability culture responds vigorously to potential failures (NMs) and views them as gifts or opportunities to address system failures.

In the surgical realm, this concept is best illustrated by the practice of a preoperative checklist that enables a state of mindfulness before embarking on a high hazard undertaking, such as a surgical procedure.[10] A more complete approach is the practice of a preoperative briefing in which a discussion occurs among members of a team regarding what problems may arise during a particular case. At the completion of the operation, a debriefing is also of value not only for determining what could have been done differently but also for discussing the planned transition toward the next phase of a patient's care. The debriefing is meant to create a reflective pause to specifically anticipate what could potentially go wrong given what has transpired up to this point. It is this collective, persistent, and watchful search for potential hazards, particularly at transition points and during periods of high technical and cognitive overload, that characterizes a high reliability surgical microsystem.[11]

Reluctance to simplify

Complex systems like a surgical environment can be unpredictable and highly nuanced. Yet, when routines set in, safe and event-free operations can lead to cutting corners, reducing resources, and eliminating key steps as waste. Simple algorithms and heuristic rules are alluring but may not take into account the nonlinear requirements of judgments, anticipation, and insights needed for excellent surgical care. This tendency seems to be amplified during times of stressed operations. A reluctance to simplify, alternatively, contributes to an enhanced understanding, especially by management, that the environment is complex, unstable, and unpredictable. A systems approach to verifying sponge and instrument count requires, for example, at minimum, a 2-person independent check and takes into account that a simple process that relies on a single person without redundancy is fraught with the possibility of error in preventing retained foreign objects.

Sensitivity to operations

HROs are highly sensitive to small deviations and interruptions in operations and allocate undivided attention to the relevant tasks affected. Unexpected events uncover loopholes in a system's defense barriers. Continuous interactivity and robust information sharing in tightly coupled systems occurs to ensure that all members of a team have a big picture view of operations. Complacency in a routine environment is a threat to maintaining sensitivity to operations. Suboptimal information sharing and a lack of awareness of other operational functions reduce redundancy and result in poor coordination. Systems are organized around the idea of creating and maintaining situational awareness by an entire team. There is an emphasis on having access to the most current and accurate information available and using it quickly in decision making particularly when unexpected deviations are detected.

Committed to resilience

The development of capabilities to recover from a failure and to contain its effects is an important characteristic of HROs. In tightly coupled systems, this resilience allows organizations to keep errors small when they occur. Hospital units exhibit resilience when they can identify and respond to smaller system failures quickly before problems escalate into significant events. To accomplish this goal they must be prepared to improvise quickly and to respond rapidly to unplanned events using preplanned routines. The inability to recover from small lapses results in brittleness, a sort of organizational failure to rescue.

Deference to expertise

Organizational units encourage decisions to be made at the front line and yield decision making to those individuals with the most expertise to fix the problem, regardless of rank. These HRO systems have developed a culture where managers and executives support the concept of deferring judgments and actions to those with the most immediately relevant knowledge and skill set. This entrusting characteristic builds immense social capital, which helps build a more honest and transparent relationship between management and clinicians.[12,13]

The hierarchical group models commonly found in health care settings contain dynamics that insist on deference given to rank and educational level among various members of the health care team. This distribution of roles, although useful during normal operations, can often be a barrier to critical decision making and information exchange during times of duress and system failure. This is not to say that coordination and other leadership tasks should not be preserved by senior leaders during these periods. In the presence of a perceived threat or an unexplained variation, however, lower ranking members of a surgical team should be able to express their concern without the risk of being subjected to ridicule or shame. Mature leaders recognize the advantage of this approach and promote relationships within teams during normal operations that allow those with the most accurate information and relevant roles to act decisively and quickly to resolve a problem. The absence of psychological safety among any member of a team can suppress potentially critical information in identifying and mitigating a threat. Edmondson[14] studied learning in interdisciplinary teams and the adoption of new technology in cardiac surgical teams, and demonstrated that the most successful teams were those with leaders who promoted speaking up as well as other coordination behaviors. Furthermore, in this study, the most effective leaders helped their teams learn by minimizing concerns about power and status differences to promote speaking up by all team members.

The relationships among the individual components of a system are critical, particularly during a catastrophic event. The robustness, resiliency, and redundancy in the physical or workflow design of these interdependencies refers to their coupling. A major distinction between high reliability theory and normal accident theory (NAT) pertains to ideas regarding the coupling between system components (**Table 1**).[15] NAT holds that accidents in complex, tightly coupled technologic systems are inevitable. Errors and failures escalate rapidly throughout a system's interdependent components.[16] Tightly coupled processes have little or no slack in this relationship.

Table 1
Comparison of the High Reliability Organizational theory and the theory of normal accidents

High Reliability Theory	Normal Accidents Theory
Accidents can be prevented through good organizational design and management.	Accidents are inevitable in complex and tightly coupled systems.
Safety is the priority organizational objective.	Safety is one of several competing values.
Redundancy enhances safety: duplication and overlap can make a reliable system out of unreliable parts.	Redundancy often causes accidents; it increases interactive complexity and opaqueness and encourages risk taking.
Decentralized decision making is needed to permit prompt and flexible field-level responses to surprises.	Organizational contradiction: decentralization is needed for complexity, but centralization is needed for tightly coupled systems.
A culture of reliability enhances safety by encouraging uniform and appropriate responses by field-level operators.	A military model of intense discipline, socialization, and isolation is incompatible with [American] democratic values.
Continuous operations, training, and simulations can create and maintain high reliability operations.	Organizations cannot train for unimagined, highly dangerous, or politically unpalatable operations.
Trial-and-error learning from accidents can be effective and can be supplemented by anticipation and simulations.	Denial of responsibility, faulty reporting, and reconstruction of history cripples learning efforts.

From Sagan SD. The limits of safety. Organizations, accidents, and nuclear weapons. Princeton (NJ): Princeton University Press; 1993. © 1993, 1995 paperback edition. *Reprinted by* permission of Princeton University Press.

As an example, the transfer of a patient from an operating room to a postanesthesia care unit is a tightly coupled process requiring a just-in-time framework of service delivery.[17] Incongruities in the magnitude, duration, and intensity of information exchange at this transition point, as reflected in postoperative orders or incomplete handoff practices, can result in critical informational gaps, creating blind spots and other opportunities for failure later in the patient journey.[18]

Highly coupled organizations value the learning opportunities provided by a continuous cascade of unsafe acts, NMs, and even full-blown adverse events because the same etiologic patterns and relationships precede both adverse events and NMs.[19,20] Only the presence or absence of recovery mechanisms determines the actual outcome. It could be argued that focusing on NM data can add significantly more value to quality improvement than a sole focus on adverse events. Schemes for reporting NMs, close calls, or sentinel (ie, warning) events have been institutionalized in aviation, nuclear power, petrochemicals, steel production, and military operations.[21,22] In health care, efforts are being made to create medical NM incident reporting systems to supplement the limited data available through mandatory reporting systems focused on preventable deaths and serious injuries.[23]

In contrast to adverse outcomes, the analysis of NMs offers several advantages: (1) NMs occur 3 to 300 times more frequently than adverse events, enabling quantitative analysis; (2) fewer barriers to data collection exist, allowing analysis of interrelationships of small failures; (3) recovery strategies can be studied to enhance proactive interventions and de-emphasize the culture of blame; (4) hindsight bias, the human tendency to see events that have already occurred as more predictable than they really were, is more effectively reduced[24]; and (5) NMs offer powerful reminders of system hazards and retard the process of forgetting to be afraid.

TEAMWORK AND HIGH RELIABILITY ORGANIZATIONS

Much of health care is performed by interdisciplinary teams—individuals with diversely specialized skills focused on a common task in a defined period of time and space (see the article by Harry C. Sax elsewhere in this issue for further exploration of this topic). These teams must respond flexibly together to contingencies and share responsibility for outcomes. This is particularly true of surgical care. Traditional specialty-centric clinical education and training are remiss in their assumption that individuals acquire adequate competencies in teamwork passively without any formal training. Moreover, the assessment practices used in selecting health care personnel do not explore the abilities of potential hires to work collaboratively or in a multidisciplinary fashion. Furthermore, performance incentives in health care are targeted at individuals and not at teams or other functional groups. With a few exceptions, risk management and liability data, morbidity and mortality conferences, and even quality improvement projects have not systematically addressed systems factors or teamwork issues. Substantial evidence suggests that teams routinely outperform individuals and are required to succeed in today's complex work arenas where information and resources are widely distributed, technology is becoming more complicated, and workload is increasing.[25,26] Nevertheless, an understanding of how medical teams contribute to HRO-like success and coordinate in real-life situations, especially during time-constrained and crises situations, remains incomplete.[27]

Surgical Teams

Teams make fewer mistakes than do individuals, especially when each team member knows his or her responsibilities as well as those of the other team members. Simply bringing individuals together to perform a specified task, however, does not automatically ensure that they will function as a team. Surgical teamwork depends on a willingness of clinicians from diverse backgrounds to cooperate toward a shared goal, to communicate, to work together effectively, and to improve. Each team member must be able to (1) anticipate the needs of the others, (2) adjust to each other's actions and to the changing environment, (3) monitor each other's activities and distribute workload dynamically, and (4) have a shared understanding of accepted processes and how events and actions should proceed.[28]

Surgical teams outperform individuals especially when performance requires multiple diverse skills, time constraints, judgment, and experience. Teams with clear goals and effective communication strategies can adjust to new information with speed and effectiveness to enhance real-time problem solving. Individual behaviors change more readily on a team because team identity is less threatened by change than individuals are. Behavioral attributes of effective teamwork, including enhanced interpersonal skills, learned as a byproduct of membership on the team, can extend to other clinical arenas. Cardiac surgical and trauma teams, among many other teams, often manifest some of these behaviors without being aware of them. Turning surgical care experts into expert surgical teams requires substantial planning and practice. There is a natural resistance to moving beyond individual roles and accountability to a team mindset. This commitment can be facilitated by (1) fostering a shared awareness of each member's tasks and role in the team through cross-training and other team training modalities; (2) training members in specific teamwork skills, such as communication, situation awareness, leadership, follower-ship, resource allocation, and adaptability; (3) conducting team training in simulated scenarios with a focus on both team behaviors and technical skills; (4) training surgical team leaders in the necessary leadership competencies to build and maintain effective teams; and (5) establishing and consistently using reliable methods of team performance evaluation and rapid feedback.[29]

Evaluating Team Performance

Assessing surgical team dynamics is a prerequisite to improving performance and increasing patient safety (**Box 1**). There is a persistent argument in the literature that team process and outcomes must be distinguished. Process is defined as the activities, strategies, responses, and behaviors used by a team during task accomplishment, whereas outcomes refer to those clinical outcomes of the patients cared for by the team.[30] Process measures are important for training when the purpose of measurement is to diagnose performance problems and to provide feedback to trainees. Until recently, the medical community has focused more on outcomes than on process. Medical educators have begun to appreciate the competencies that define an effective team process.[31] The key to clinical alignment is to identify and measure processes that are directly related to patient outcomes (eg, successful resuscitation). Measurement tools must be reliable and valid, and they must distinguish between individual and team-level deficiencies (**Table 2**).[32–34] Perhaps most importantly, the results of the assessment must be translatable into specific feedback to team members that can help enhance their team performance.[35]

CLINICAL MICROSYSTEMS

Several models of care delivery have emerged as health care institutions face challenges in providing safe, reliable, and effective health care in a complex regulatory and financially burdened environment.[36] Many organizations have struggled to design operational units that can best incorporate reliable and service-oriented performance into their daily work. Microsystems, based on work of intelligent enterprises by Quinn[37] applies systems thinking to organizational design and represent the smallest replicable organizational unit of change. Quinn studied companies that achieved consistent growth, high quality, and high margins as well as exceptional reputations with their customers. He found that these smallest replicable units were the key to implementing effective strategy, leveraging information technology, and embedding

---

Box 1
Questions to ask when assessing a surgical team's performance

- Is the team the right size and composition?
- Are there adequate levels of complementary skills?
- Is there a shared goal for the team?
- Does everyone understand the team goals?
- Has a set of performance goals been agreed on?
- Do the team members hold one another accountable for the group's results?
- Are there shared protocols and performance ground rules?
- Is there mutual respect and trust between team members?
- Do team members communicate effectively?
- Do team members know and appreciate each other's roles and responsibilities?
- When one team member is absent or not able to perform the assigned tasks, are other team members able to pitch in or help appropriately?

Table 2
Individual and team-level training strategies

	Definition	Level
Assertiveness Training	Uses behavioral modeling techniques to demonstrate both assertive and nonassertive behaviors; provides multiple practice and feedback opportunities for trainees	Individual
Metacognitive Training	Targets trainee's executive monitoring and self-regulatory cognitive processes for development; training develops metacognitive skills that regulate cognitive abilities, such as inductive and deductive reasoning	Individual
Stress Exposure Training	Provides information regarding links between stressors, trainee affect, and performance; provides coping strategies to help trainees deal with stressors	Individual and team

Data from Refs.[32–34]

other performance-enhancing practices into the service delivery process. Health care microsystems consist of a small group of people who provide care to a defined set of patients and for a particular purpose, such as a surgical ICU (**Table 3**). They have both clinical and business aims, tightly coupled processes, and a shared information environment. Clinical, service, and financial outcomes are measured systematically and with a view toward continuous improvement.

Real-time collection, analysis, and sharing of information are key features of these groups that generally function within a larger organization providing a clear financial, regulatory, and legal framework. A microsystem's developmental journey toward maturation and improved performance entails 5 stages of growth (**Box 2**).[38] The role of senior leaders in a microsystem is to look for ways in which the meso-organization, working within the macro-organization's legal and regulatory framework, connects with and facilitates the work of the microsystem. The meso-organization, in turn, supports the needs and facilitates coordination among varying microsystems to accomplish the organization's overarching goals. The clinical microsystem approach emphasizes identifying and promoting the strengths of both the team and individuals. It maintains a focus on continuous improvement rather than externally imposed targets and initiatives that members think do not directly have an impact on their work. Many organizations using this approach have demonstrated high levels of staff

Table 3
The 5 essential goals (5 Ps) of the microsystem

5 Ps	What are the Implications for Effective Microsystem Functioning?
Purpose	What is the purpose of the clinical microsystem and how does that purpose fit within the overall vision?
Patients	Who are the people served by the microsystem?
Professionals	Who are the staff who work together in the microsystem?
Processes	What are the care-giving and support processes the microsystem uses to provide care and services?
Patterns	What are the patterns that characterize microsystem functioning?

From Barach P, Johnson JK. Understanding the complexity of redesigning care around clinical microsystem. Qual Saf Health Care 2006;15(Suppl 1);10–6; with permission.

Box 2
Clinical microsystems: 5 stages of growth

- Awareness as an interdependent group with the capacity to make changes
- Connecting routine daily work to the high purpose of benefiting patients
- Responding successfully to strategic challenges
- Measuring performance as a system
- Juggling improvements while taking care of patients

Data from Batalden PB, Nelson EC, Edwards WH, et al. Microsystems in health care: part 9. Developing small clinical units to attain peak performance. Jt Comm J Qual Saf 2003; 29(11):575–85.

satisfaction, an enhanced level of empowerment, and increased commitment toward established goals as well as a passion for continuous learning and innovation.[39]

In addition, the microsystem incorporates the experience and perceptions of patients and their families in the strategic development to deliver the most desirable service from the point of view of the end user.[40] A surgical microsystem can involve, for example, a pediatric cardiac surgical team that includes the corresponding critical care team, wards, or perhaps a large surgical critical care unit providing services in a defined geographic space.[41,42] The microsystem will include patients and their family members given that there is a convergence of purpose in a patient's full recovery.

Microsystems and Patient Safety

Safety is a fundamental property of the microsystem. It can only be achieved through thoughtful and systematic application of a broad array of process, equipment, organization, supervision, training, simulation, and teamwork changes. Characteristics of high-performing microsystems—leadership, organizational support, staff focus, education and training, interdependence, patient focus, community and market focus, performance results, process improvement, and information and information technology—can be linked to specific design concepts and actions to enhance patient safety in microsystems.[43]

Leadership and Patient Safety

Leaders directly contribute to the performance of microsystems. The role of senior leadership within an organization changes in scope and focus and is more externally focused provided that each microsystem in an organization has a tight alignment with the overall mission and vision of the organization.[36] The result is that each microsystem possesses the flexibility to achieve its specific performance goals while ensuring the safety and reliability of the care it provides. This strategy allows for the creation of each unit's climate of safety. Previous work in the field of organizational behavior, highlighted by the Michigan Keystone ICU Project to reduce central line infections, have demonstrated that positive deviance is well at work at the unit level, and that unit-based culture can have an impact on those other microsystems with which they interface.[44] Equally important, Dixon Woods and colleagues[45] have demonstrated that the checklist's key impact was to shape a culture of commitment by leadership and clinicians to doing better in practice around reducing central line infections as the major driver for success.

RECOMMENDATIONS AND 6 PRINCIPLES FOR DESIGNING SAFE SURGICAL MICROSYSTEMS

Based on the authors' experience with multiple microsystems across diverse settings and with an understanding and interpretation of the safety literature, several safety principles that can be used as a framework for embedding patient safety concepts within clinical surgical microsystems are discussed.[46]

Principle 1—Errors are Human Nature and will Happen Because Humans are not Infallible

Errors are not synonymous with negligence. Medicine's ethos of infallibility leads wrongly to a culture that sees mistakes as an individual problem or weakness and remedies them with blame and punishment instead of looking for the multiple contributing factors that can only be solved by improving systems.

Principle 2—the Microsystem is the Optimal Unit of Intervention, Analysis, and Training

Microsystem staff can be trained to include safety principles in their daily work through rehearsing scenarios, simulation, and role-playing. The goal is for a microsystem to behave like a robust HRO, that is, preoccupied with the possibility for failure or chronic unease about safety breaches.

Principle 3—Design Systems to Identify, Prevent, Absorb, and Mitigate Errors

Identify errors by establishing effective sustainable reporting systems that encourage and support transparency, freedom from punitive actions, and empowering workers to feel comfortable speaking up, even if speaking up means that they challenge the authority gradient. Design work, technology, and work practices to uncover, mitigate, or attenuate the consequences of error. There are many ways to reduce the impact of errors by simplifying systems and processes. For example, tools, such as checklists, flow sheets, and ticklers, to reduce reliance on memory all address deficiencies in vigilance and memory. Improve access to information and information technology. Systems must be designed to absorb a certain amount of error without harm to patients. Key buffers might include time lapses (built-in delays, when appropriate, to verify information before proceeding), redundancy, force functions, and so forth.

Principle 4—Create a Culture of Safety

A safety culture is one that recognizes that the cornerstone to making health care safer is a transparent climate that supports reporting errors, NMs, and adverse events; feeds this information back quickly and clearly to clinicians; and holds clinicians accountable for their actions (**Box 3**).[47]

Principle 5—Talk to and Listen to Patients

Patients have much to say about surgical safety and how they can add to the resilience of a system. Embrace and celebrate storytelling by patients and clinicians—that is where safety is made and breached and much learning occurs. When a patient is harmed by health care, all details of the event pertaining to the patient should be disclosed with the patient and/or the family (see the article by Eaves-Leanos and Dunn elsewhere in this issue for further exploration of this topic). Elements of disclosure include[48]:

- A prompt and compassionate explanation of what is understood about what happened and the probable effects

---

Box 3
Characteristics of safety-focused teams

- Ongoing organizational learning
- Transparency in discussing errors
- Respect for the value and response to NMs
- Supporting communication among team members
- Members function as part of a team
- Culture that supports questioning the leader or more senior team members
- Prioritizing task demands
- Aligning occupational cultures
- Establishing and maintaining clear roles and goals
- Experienced team members
- Adequate number of dedicated surgical team members
- Establishing and maintaining consistent supportive organizational infrastructure
- Leaders with the right stuff
- Peer-to-peer assessment tools

Data from Barach P, Weinger M. Trauma team performance. In: Wilson WC, Grande CM, Hoyt DB, editors. Trauma: emergency resuscitation and perioperative anesthesia management, vol. 1. New York: Marcel Dekker; 2007. p. 101–13. ISBN: 10-0-8247-2916-6.

- Assurance that a full analysis will take place to reduce the likelihood of a similar event happening to another patient
- Follow-up based on the analysis and an apology to the patient and family

Principle 6—Integrate Practices from Human Factors Engineering into Surgical Microsystem Functioning

Design patient-centered health care environments that are based on human factors principles and constraints; design for human cognitive failings and the impact of performance-shaping factors—fatigue, poor lighting, noisy settings, and so forth.

SUMMARY

This article explores the applicability of high reliability and microsystems theories to the surgical environment. Safety is a fundamental property of both. It might be argued that improving safety in surgical systems does not require an entire restructuring of organizations and workflow; however, despite intense attention to this subject over the past decade, incremental improvement in safety has not been forthcoming with the existing models of care. Moreover, current systems have failed to address the patients' overall needs.

Health care institutions continue to face challenges in providing safe patient care in increasingly complex and demanding technical, organizational, and regulatory environments. Both high reliability theory and clinical microsystems provide conceptual and practical frameworks for approaching the delivery of safe care. Although many ambiguities and conflicts arise from the implementation of these theoretic constructs, they should guide the development of work processes and stimulate innovation in designing ways to provide safe and effective care within health care systems.

Organizing surgical care around the pursuit of safety as an overarching priority is a professional obligation for all members of the health care team. This goal can be accomplished by organizing around and shaping a culture focused on reliable performance but requires substantial investments in human capital. Readily accessible communication and information sharing are essential components for creating high reliability. A clinical microsystem concept involving surgical personnel can be an effective vehicle for achieving these goals.

Facilitating the design of systems to identify, prevent, absorb, and mitigate errors can provide remarkable opportunities for improving safety. The authors think these concepts are complementary and can be synergistic. Each can embed safety into surgical processes, not as an add-on value but as an integral element. Incorporating these broad concepts provides an ideal framework for capturing opportunities to improve surgical care. It is in this context that movement toward safer care can take place.

REFERENCES

1. Berlow EL, Dunne JA, Martinez ND, et al. Simple prediction of interaction strengths in complex food webs. Proceedings of the National Academy of Sciences 2009;106:187–219.
2. Weick KE, Sutcliffe KM. Managing the unexpected: assuring high performance in an age of complexity. New York: John Wiley and Sons, Inc; 2001.
3. Woods D. How to design a safety organization: test case for resilience engineering. In: Hollnagel E, Woods DD, Leveson N, editors. Resilience engineering: concepts and precepts. United Kingdom: Ashgate Publishing; 2006. p. 315–24.
4. Hollnagel E, Woods DD, Leveson N. Resilience engineering: concepts and precepts. United Kingdom: Ashgate Publishing Limited; 2006.
5. Wears RL, Perry S, Anders S, et al. Resilience in the emergency department. In: Hollnagel E, Nemeth C, Dekker SWA, editors. Resilience engineering perspectives 1: remaining sensitive to the possibility of failure. Aldershot (UK): Ashgate; 2008. p. 193–209.
6. Weick KE, Sutcliffe KM, Obstfeld D. Organizing for high reliability: processes of collective mindfulness. In: Staw B, Sutton R, editors. Research in Organizational Behavior, vol. 21. Greenwich (CT): JAI; 1999. p. 81–123.
7. Reason JT. Human error. New York: Cambridge University Press; 1990.
8. Reason JT, Carthey J, de Leval MR. Diagnosing "vulnerable system syndrome": an essential prerequisite to effective risk management. Qual Health Care 2001; 10(Suppl 2):ii21–5.
9. Vaughn D. The challenger launch decision: risky technology, culture, and deviance at NASA. Chicago: The University of Chicago Press; 1996.
10. Haynes AB, Weiser TG, Berry WR, et al, Safe Surgery Saves Lives Study Group. A surgical safety checklist to reduce morbidity and mortality in a global population. N Engl J Med 2009;360(5):491–9.
11. Weick KE, Roberts KH. Collective mind in organizations: heedful interrelating on flight decks. Adm Sci Q 1993;38:357–81.
12. Zohar D. Safety climate in industrial organizations; theoretical and applied implications. J Appl Psychol 1980;65:96–102.
13. Sexton J, Helmreich R, Thomas E. Error, stress and teamwork in medicine and aviation: cross sectional surveys. BMJ 2000;320:745–9.
14. Edmondson AC. Speaking up in the operating room: how team leaders promote learning in interdisciplinary action teams. Journal of Management Studies 2003; 40:1419–52.

15. Sagan SD. The limits of safety. Organizations, accidents, and nuclear weapons. Princeton (NJ): Princeton University Press; 1993.
16. Tamuz M, Harrison MI. Improving patient safety in hospitals: contributions of high-reliability theory and normal accident theory. Health Serv Res 2006;41(4 Pt 2): 1654–76.
17. Catchpole KR, de Leval MR, McEwan A, et al. Patient handover from surgery to intensive care: using Formula 1 pit-stop and aviation models to improve safety and quality. Paediatr Anaesth 2007;17:470–8.
18. Catchpole K, Sellers R, Goldman A, et al. Patient handovers within the hospital: translating knowledge from motor racing to healthcare. Qual Saf Health Care 2010;19:318–22.
19. Gambino R, Mallon O. Near misses—an untapped database to find root causes. Lab Report 1991;13:41–4.
20. March JG, Sproull LS, Tamuz M. Learning from samples of one or fewer. Organ Sci 1991;2:1–3.
21. Reynard WD, Billings CE, Cheney ES, et al. The development of the NASA aviation safety reporting system. NASA Aeronautics and Space Administration, Scientific and Technical Information Branch; 1986. NASA Reference Publication 1114. Available at: http://www-afo.arc.nasa.gov/ASRS/callback.html. Accessed December 4, 2011.
22. Ives G. Near miss reporting pitfalls for nuclear plants. In: Van der Shaff TW, Lucas DA, Hale AR, editors. Near miss reporting as a safety tool. Oxford (UK): Butterworth and Heineman; 1991.
23. Carroll J. Incident reviews in High-hazard industries: sense making and learning under ambiguity and accountability. Ind Environ Crisis Q 1995;9(2):175–97.
24. Barach P, Small SD. Reporting and preventing medical mishaps: lessons from non-medical near miss reporting systems. BMJ 2000;320:753–63.
25. Bradford DL, Cohen AR. Managing for excellence: the guide to developing high performance contemporary organizations. New York: John Wiley & Sons; 1984.
26. Katzenbach JR, Smith DK. The wisdom of teams: creating the high performance organization. Cambridge (MA): Harvard Business School Press; 1993.
27. Barach P. Team based risk modification program to make health care safer. Theor Issues Ergon Sci 2007;8:481–94.
28. Barach P, Johnson J. Team based learning in microsystems—an organizational framework for success. Technology, Instruction, Cognition and Learning 2006; 3:307–21.
29. Baker D, Salas E, Barach P, et al. The relation between teamwork and patient safety. In: Carayon P, editor. Handbook of human factors and ergonomics in health care and patient safety. New Jersey: Lawrence Erlbaum Associates, Inc; 2006. p. 259–71.
30. Lilford R, Chilton PJ, Hemming K, et al. Evaluating policy and service interventions: a methodological classification. BMJ 2010;341:c4413.
31. Baker DP, Gustafson S, Beaubien JM, et al. Programs, tools, and products. AHRQ Publication No. 05-0021-4. Medical team training programs in health care. Advances in patient safety: from research to implementation, vol. 4. Rockville (MD): Agency for Healthcare Research and Quality; 2005.
32. Smith-Jentsch KA, Zeisig RL, Acton B, et al. Team dimensional training. In: Cannon-Bowers JA, Salas E, editors. Making decisions under stress: implications for individual and team training. Washington, DC: American Psychological Association; 1998. p. 271–97.

33. Jentsch F. Metacognitive training for junior team members: solving the "copilot's catch-22." Unpublished doctoral dissertation. Orlando (FL): University of Central Florida; 1997.

34. Driskell JE, Johnston JH. Stress exposure training. In: Cannon-Bowers JA, Salas E, editors. Making decisions under stress—implications for individual and team training. Washington, DC: American Psychological Association; 1998. p. 191–217.

35. Performance measurement in teams. Team training series, book 2. Orlando (FL): Naval Air Warfare Center Training Systems Division.

36. Mohr J, Barach P, Cravero J, et al. Microsystems in health care. Jt Comm J Qual Saf 2003;29:401–8.

37. Quinn JB. Intelligent enterprise: a knowledge and service based paradigm for industry. New York: Free Press; 1992.

38. Batalden PB, Nelson EC, Edewards WH, et al. Microsystems in health care: part 9. Developing small clinical units to attain peak performance. Jt Comm J Qual Saf 2003;29(11):575–85.

39. Williams I, Dickinson H, Robinson S, et al. Clinical microsystems and the NHS: a sustainable method for improvement? J Health Organ Manag 2009;23(1): 119–32.

40. Reis MD, Scott SD, Rempel GR. Including parents in the evaluation of clinical microsystems in the neonatal intensive care unit. Adv Neonatal Care 2009;9(4): 174–9.

41. Schraagen JM, Schouten A, Smit M, et al. Improving methods for studying teamwork in cardiac surgery. Qual Saf Health Care 2010;19:1–6.

42. Schraagen JM, Schouten T, Smit M, et al. A prospective study of paediatric cardiac surgical microsystems: assessing the relationships between non-routine events, teamwork and patient outcomes. BMJ Qual Saf 2011;20(7): 599–603.

43. Barach P, Johnson J. Assessing risk and harm in the clinical microsystem: a systematic approach to patient safety. In: Sollecito W, Johnson J, editors. Continuous quality improvement in health care: theory, implementations, and applications. 4th edition. Jones and Bartlett; 2011. p. 249–74.

44. Pronovost P, Wu A, Dorman T, et al. Building safety into ICU care. J Crit Care 2002;17:78–85.

45. Dixon Woods M, Bosk CL, Aveling E, et al. Explaining Michigan: developing an ex post theory of a quality improvement program. Milbank Q A Multidisciplinary Journal of Population and Health Policy 2011;89:167–205.

46. Johnson J, Barach P. Safety: mindfulness for increased reliability and safety. In: Nelson E, Batalden P, Godfrey M, editors. Clinical microsystem action guide. 3rd edition. Hanover (NH): Trustees of Dartmouth College; 2010. p. 89–100.

47. Barach P, Johnson JK. Understanding the complexity of redesigning care around clinical microsystem. Qual Saf Health Care 2006;15(Suppl 1):10–6.

48. Cantor M, Barach P, Derse A, et al. Disclosing adverse events to patients. Jt Comm J Qual Patient Saf 2005;31:5–12.

Building High-Performance Teams in the Operating Room

Harry C. Sax, MD, MHCM

KEYWORDS

• Patient safety • Team dynamics • Communication

This is a democracy—everyone votes and I decide.
—Attributed to one of my chief residents

As surgeons, we were trained in not only personal responsibility for our patients but also leadership of teams. The hierarchy was clearly defined, and teams were a relatively homogeneous collection of surgical residents, medical students, and perhaps a nurse practitioner. We learned how to function in the operating room (OR) by observing attending surgeons and tried to assess the characteristics of those who seemed successful in engaging all those present. Other disciplines involved in the same patient care had different experiences and perspectives. What we perceive as good teamwork and communication are seen by others as less than adequate. In a study of OR and ICU teams, 84% of anesthesiologists and 94% of intensivists felt that junior team members should be able to question the decisions of more senior members. Only 55% of attending surgeons and 58% of surgical residents agreed. Nurses' response patterns mimicked those of anesthesiologists and intensivists. Similarly, surgeons were less likely to acknowledge the effects of personal stress and fatigue on performance.[1] Is it any wonder that with different expectations and perceptions, effective team building is a challenge?

LEARNING FROM THOSE THAT DO IT WELL

In the business community, the financial viability and survival of an organization is dependent on delivering high-quality goods and services in response to customers' needs.[2] Bringing together teams with members that have different skills and personalities involves several steps for success:

1. The creation of a shared belief in the value of the team and of the mission
2. Setting clear and achievable goals

The author has nothing to disclose.
Department of Surgery, Cedars-Sinai Medicine Clinical Transformation Initiative, Cedars-Sinai Medical Center, 8700 Beverly Boulevard, NT 8215, Los Angeles, CA 90048, USA
E-mail address: saxh@cshs.org

3. Ensuring a desire to work with others to achieve the goals
4. Recognizing the value of all team members, no matter where they sit in the hierarchy
5. Instilling in individuals an awareness of how valuable their own contribution is to the team
6. Rewarding desirable team behavior in tangible and nontangible ways.

What makes team building in ORs a challenge:

1. Although everyone in an OR is drawn by patient care, motivations are different. Surgeons want to treat the illness or injury, have built a relationship with patients, and will care for pateints after leaving the surgical suite. Anesthesiologists are tasked with acutely maintaining hemodynamic functioning during an active insult while providing medications that are inherently toxic. Nurses have a strong identity as patient advocates and protectors. In addition, they are saddled with multiple policies and procedures that may put them at crossed purposes with others in the room. Based on outside responsibilities, there may also be time considerations, and some team members have the option of being replaced during the procedure should they need to leave. Finally, students want to learn the techniques of their mentors and try not to get in the way.
2. The goal is to provide patients with optimal safe care; not everyone is aligned to that goal. Production pressures and outside responsibilities divert individuals from focusing on patients and induces tunnel vision that limits efforts to a single task.
3. We were judged and rewarded for our individual achievements. Nobody ever got into medical or nursing school by being a C student yet a great team player. In other fields, the ability to function in a team environment is taught and rewarded.
4. By being trained in a hierarchy, it is difficult to recognize the value of each individual independent of their level. Yet one of the most hierarchical of all institutions, the US Marine Corps, is an example of superb team functioning. The Marines create an identity and culture that recognizes an individual's skills and instills in each member the ability to seek ways to adapt those skills to the betterment of the team.[3]
5. A well-known chief of surgery once said, "I don't give compliments. Perfection in patient care is expected—everything else needs an explanation." An appropriate goal to be sure, yet could the same results be achieved incrementally with reward and recognition? By creating all-or-nothing thinking, are we optimizing our ability to improve the system?

DEVELOPING THE TEAM—DOES EVERYONE KNOW THE GOAL?

Although the concept of the OR team centers around the acute time when a patient is having a procedure, many groups function in support of that patient. The efficiency and effectiveness of room turnover and supply availability can affect the operative team by reducing fatigue and stress as well as eliminating extra handoffs that occur when scheduled cases run late. There is a tendency to focus only on a specific assigned role without seeing how our contributions affect the overall process. Effective organizations help individual employees understand their role in the overall mission and invest the resources to orient and support those behaviors. Effective organizations seek input from those on the front line, and engage them in solving problems and optimizing flow. Trust is established by sharing data and providing feedback.

OK, WHAT ARE SOME PRACTICAL INTERVENTIONS?

The following suggestions in and of themselves do not create effective teams. They may, however, improve communication and focus goal alignments.

1. Establish clear expectations for team member behaviors and orient new employees to institutional goals and culture. New members to an operative team often feel excluded as to the nuances of how established groups work together. The normal onboarding process is often limited to a brief explanation of how to complete forms and where to find scrubs. A clear review of conflict management, the need for error reporting, and a safe place to express concerns are vital.
2. Align incentives with desired behaviors. Teams in outpatient surgicenters know that if they are efficient, they go home early and are paid for the full day. In other organizations, finishing early means being assigned another case, without additional compensation. Hospital contracts with specialties like anesthesiology can focus on mutually agreed-on goals, based on sharing data and exceeding national benchmarks.
3. Create multidisciplinary process improvement teams coupled with expanded morbidity and mortality conference. Participants should include surgeons, nurses, anesthesiologist, pathologists, radiologists, and critical care Physicians. The presence of all disciplines emphasizes interdependence in the care of patients. With good facilitation, the normal finger pointing seen in seeking to assign blame can be replaced by constructive discussion of how to improve care.
4. Solicit active feedback to suggestions for change. Team members feel empowered when they feel that their suggestions are heard. Establish a suggestion box, and post all the suggestions, with the administrator assigned to deal with them, followed by the findings and resolution.
5. Establish friendly competition among teams—if the issue is turnover time, have monthly goals established and post the results in real time. The winning team gets recognition by a party or paid time off.
6. Rapidly and consistently address disruptive behavior—team training, checklists, and policies and procedures provide a framework for team functioning. Open communication is predicated on trust, and team members can shut down communication by being demeaning, passive aggressive, or openly cynical. It is the responsibility of leadership to intervene quickly when observing or learning of incidents. In many cases, this is a one-time event, often stimulated by outside influences. Recurrent episodes, however, should be addressed through appropriate counseling, remediation, and monitoring. In situations where there is a unionized workforce, early involvement by the shop steward and human resources is vital. Physicians can be more problematic. There are specific bylaws established by the medical staff, and these provide progressive guidance. Should pressure be brought to bear by administrators concerned with the financial contribution of the individual, appropriate involvement by the chief medical officer is vital, with eventual involvement of the chief executive officer. Great leaders know the importance of setting expectations and sending consistent messages. Organizations' true key values are measured by making the right decision, even if it costs market share.
7. Hire for attitude, train for aptitude. Southwest Airlines is widely cited as an organization that has defined a culture and expects those who join to understand and commit to it. During the pilot selection process, shuttle bus drivers are queried as to how they were treated by the candidates. Southwest realized we can all put on a good game face when we know we are being watched.[4] Data have shown

that behavioral issues in medical school and training auger future difficulties in practice. This is not to say that these individuals should not be brought on staff.[5] Credentialling committees should probe more deeply into whether applicant with past behavioral difficulties have gained insight into their strengths and weaknesses.

8. Identify informal leaders, even if they are not in leadership positions. Every organization has members who are respected by others and can be thought of as leaders. These champions, if embraced, can help overcome resistance to change and model behaviors that encourage communication and inclusiveness. This should include those who have a tendency to challenge administration.

9. Assure that there is institutional support for team building initiatives with prompt responses to identified issues. Despite a decade of work on the use of team training in the OR environment, few clear outcomes can be tied to the initiatives. The most visible success was a report from the medical team training (MTT) program at the San Francisco VA Medical Center. The program included 4 components: a 1-day interactive learning session for all operative staff on the principles of crew resource management, preoperative briefings and postoperative debriefings using standardized checklists, and, most uniquely, a multidisciplinary MTT executive committee that identifies potential systems issues. During the debriefing, held in the OR immediately after surgery, the team assigned a numeric score to indicate how the case went. There was prompt follow-up and feedback of findings to the teams. This labor-intensive program reviewed more than 4000 cases. The MTT committee resolved many systems problems, such as equipment ordering, stocking, and blood gas protocols as well as getting inpatient medications into the OR for intraoperative use. A subsequent survey showed that 80% of staff thought the program had improved patient safety in the OR, approximately 75% believed it improved the OR atmosphere, and almost 60% thought there was better follow-up of OR issues. Staff attitudes improved significantly after MTT on 5 of 6 domains on the Safety Attitudes Questionnaire, except for stress recognition.[6]

Other studies of team training have shown only increased awareness and perceived empowerment without these types of objective changes.[7,8] The Department of Veterans Affairs environment has a different financial and structural organization, however, than not-for-profit community hospitals of academic medical centers.

THERE IS NO EASY FIX AND THE RETURN ON INVESTMENT IS TOUGH TO QUANTIFY

We have been trained to analyze a patient's medical issues, confirm our impressions with objective testing, and intervene surgically if the benefits outweigh the risks. During a procedure, specific steps are performed and modifications made in the plan based on new findings. Postoperatively, we monitor recovery and treat complications should they arise. The building of effective teams can follow a similar pattern while recognizing that diagnosing a pathology requires a different set of skills, response to interventions may be delayed and hard to quantify, and measures of success will be in new areas, such as decreased employee turnover, increased error reporting due to improved trust, disagreements that are welcomed as a chance to look at new perspectives, and a sense that each of us is part of something bigger.[2] Chief financial officers will not see changes in service line contribution margins until they realize that 4 cases are being done during a day that normally could only accommodate 3 and employee and patient satisfaction scores (soon to be publicly reported) are up.

Everybody can vote, and there will still be leaders who will have ultimate responsibility for outcomes. Perhaps, however, those leaders will make better decisions knowing they are heading a cohesive team.

REFERENCES

1. Sexton JB, Thomas EJ, Helmreich RL. Error, stress, and teamwork in medicine and aviation: cross sectional surveys. BMJ 2000;320(7237):745–9.
2. Lencioni P. The five dysfunctions of a team. San Francisco: Jossey Bass; 2002.
3. Peterson GI. For corps and country; building the next generation of Marines. Available at: www.navyleague.org. Accessed July 22, 2011.
4. Taylor W. How do you know a great person when you see one? Harvard Business review blogs. Available at: http://blogs.hbr.org/taylor/2011/07/how_do_you_know_a_great_person.html?cm_sp=most_widget-_-default-_-. Accessed July 22, 2011.
5. Papadakis MA, Teherani A, Banach MA, et al. Disciplinary action by medical boards and prior behavior in medical school. N Engl J Med 2005;353(25):2673–82.
6. Wolf FA, Way LW, Stewart L. The efficacy of medical team training: improved team performance and decreased operating room delays: a detailed analysis of 4863 cases. Ann Surg 2010;252(3):477–83 [discussion: 483–5].
7. Sax HC, Brown P, Mayewski RJ, et al. Can aviation-based team training elicit sustainable behavioral change? Arch Surg 2009;144(12):1133–7.
8. Gore DC, Powell JM, Baer JG, et al. Crew resource management improved perception of patient safety in the operating room. Am J Med Qual 2010;25(1):60–3.

Human Factors and Operating Room Safety

Andrew W. ElBardissi, MD, MPH[a,b,]*, Thoralf M. Sundt, MD[c]

KEYWORDS

• Human factors • Operating room • Safety

There have been remarkable reductions in patient morbidity and mortality after surgical procedures over the preceding decades; however, adverse events still occur even among some low-risk patients. In many cases, surgical errors likely contribute in at least some measure to these outcomes. Historically, surgical outcomes have been attributed primarily to the technical skills of the surgeon and the medical condition and comorbidities of the patients. In general, "once patient outcomes (usually mortality) have been adjusted for patient risk factors, the remaining variance is presumed to be explained by individual surgical skill."[1] Hence, when things go wrong or surgical errors are made, it is logical from this human-centered perspective to question the particular surgeon's competency or aptitude. This is the unspoken basis of individual surgeon rankings in public reporting.

In contrast, a human factors approach recognizes that human error is often the result of a combination of both individual surgeon factors and work system factors. Specifically, the Systems Engineering Initiative to Patient Safety (SEIPS) model is based on recognition that, in addition to surgical skill, performance and outcomes are also affected by such factors as teamwork and communication, the physical working environment, technology/tool design, task and workload factors, and organizational variables. According to this perspective, errors are the natural consequences (not causes) of the systemic breakdown among the myriad work system factors affecting performance.[2] Consequently, patient safety programs are likely to be most effective when they intervene at specific failure points within the system

Supported by the Agency for Health Care Research Quality NRSA Grant 1F32HS019190 and the Arthur and Tracy Cabot Fellowship at Brigham and Women's Hospital and the Center for Surgery and Public Health.

[a] Division of Cardiac Surgery, Brigham and Women's Hospital, Harvard Medical School, 75 Francis Street, Boston, MA 02115, USA
[b] Department of Surgery, Brigham and Women's Hospital and the Center for Surgery and Public Health, Harvard Medical School, 75 Francis Street, Boston, MA 02115, USA
[c] Division of Cardiac Surgery, Massachusetts General Hospital, Harvard Medical School, 55 Fruit Street, Boston, MA 02114, USA
* Corresponding author. Division of Cardiac Surgery, Brigham and Women's Hospital, Harvard Medical School, 75 Francis Street, Boston, MA 02115.
E-mail address: aelbardissi@partners.org

rather than focusing exclusively on the competency of the individual who committed the error.[3]

Historically, most data concerning systemic factors that affect patient safety in the operating room (OR) have come from anecdotal and sentinel event reports, which often lack details concerning the specific nature of the systemic problems that affect surgical performance.[3] However, in recent years, a growing number of published studies have used prospective data collection methods, such as ethnographic and direct observation, to identify empirically the real-time dynamics of work system factors in the OR and their impact on patient safety.[4,5] Although the complexities of surgical care demand further research to fully understand the pathogenesis of surgical errors, the results of these prospective studies have begun to identify opportunities and interventions for improving surgical performance and patient outcomes. The efficacy of only a few of these interventions has been tested, and it is unlikely that any single intervention alone has a major impact on surgical care; however, most recommendations emerging from this body of research are grounded in empirical data. When considered together they provide an opportunity to develop comprehensive intervention strategies for addressing a wide variety of work system factors that affect surgical performance and patient safety in the OR.

This article reviews previous research on the impact of work system factors on surgical care. Specifically, the discussion highlights research pertaining to the following components of surgical care: (1) the physical OR environment, (2) teamwork and communication, (3) tools and technology, (4) tasks and workload, and (5) organizational processes.

THE OR ENVIRONMENT

Although most surgeons have become impervious to the complexity of the OR environment, there are numerous environmental factors that could potentially affect surgical performance. These factors include the general OR layout and clutter,[6] as well as ambient factors such as noise,[5] lighting,[7] motion/vibration, and temperature. Among these factors, OR layout and noise have received most of the attention in the literature, and accordingly are the main focus here. However, this focus does not imply that the others are unimportant.

OR Layout

Congestion because of the location of equipment and displays, as well as the disarray of wires, tubes, and lines (known as the spaghetti syndrome), is a common scenario in the OR.[8] Consequently, movement by members of the surgical team is often obstructed, wiring is difficult to access and maintain, and the risk of accidental disconnection of devices and human error are increased, all of which heighten the threat to patient safety.[9] In addition, the location of workstations and the placement of equipment relative to the surgical table can hinder communication and coordination among team members. For example, in an unpublished study of perfusionists in cardiac surgery, we identified that the perfusionist's location behind the surgeon as well as the various components of the cardiopulmonary bypass (CPB) machine that physically separated the perfusionists from the surgical table significantly hindered team performance. One of the principal problems cause by this OR layout was the inability of the perfusionists to see what was happening at the surgical field. This situation made it difficult for the perfusionist to coordinate their actions with the surgeon. As workarounds, perfusionists often anticipated the surgeon's needs using the passage of time and inferences made from the movements of surgical personnel at the table.

Similarly, the surgeon was unable to observe the actions of the perfusionist. Consequently, this OR layout and configuration often led to poor coordination of activities that subsequently disrupted the surgical flow of the operation.

A variety of recommendations for addressing the spaghetti syndrome have been proposed, including better utilization of ceiling space, such as ceiling-mounted columns that descend to the team on request and return to their place after use. Others include color-coding and arranging cables in unique patterns on the ceiling for easier identification.[6] The area under the operating table has been identified as an unused, vacant space for placing or storing equipment. The elimination of wiring through the use of wireless technology has also been proposed. A recent study[6] of electronic medical devices in the operating theater and intensive care environments indicated that Bluetooth communication did not interfere with or change the function of the medical devices and argued that the utilization of wireless technology would not only eliminate clutter and the potential for confusion and errors but would also allow equipment to be arranged in a flexible manner in the different operating theaters according to the specific operation being performed or the needs and preferences of the surgical team. However, such flexibility or variability in OR layout may not always be beneficial. Brogmus and colleagues[8] have argued that "although the needs in ORs vary according to the procedures performed, there is a good argument to be made for making the layout of ORs consistent so that efficiency is improved. For example, a consistent OR layout will have clean-up supplies on the same shelf, communication equipment in the same location, and the information monitor on the same boom. This also will reduce wasted time and, potentially, patient-threatening errors."

Although the benefits of standardization versus flexibility have long been debated, there are general principles that can be followed when determining the arrangement of components within the OR suite. These principles include (1) the importance principle (components and equipment that are vital to the achievement of a procedure or task should be placed in convenient locations); (2) the frequency of use principle (components and equipment that are frequently used during the completion of a procedure or task should be located in close proximity and be easily accessible); (3) the function principle (components, equipment, or information/displays that serve the same function or are commonly used together to make decisions or complete a task should be placed in similar locations or close to one another), and (4) the sequence of use principle (during completion of a procedure or task, certain tools and technology may be consistently used in a set sequence or order and should therefore be arranged in a manner to facilitate this process). These principles are not always independent and may even conflict when being used to make decisions regarding the rearrangement of components in the OR suite. Component location may also interfere with face-to-face communication among surgical staff or disrupt the traffic flow or movement of personnel in the OR. Consequently, considerable research is needed to collect and combine appropriate sources of data, including task analysis, anthropometric, and architectural data before specific recommendations can be made for redesigning a particular cardiac surgery OR suite.

Noise in the OR

In addition to layout and clutter, the OR environment is full of noise and distractions that can hinder the ability of the surgeon and other team members to fully concentrate on the task at hand. Noise is generally defined as auditory stimuli that bear no informational relationship to the completion of the immediate task. A recent study[5] of noise levels in the OR found that the average maximum noise level for an operation was more than 80 dB, with absolute maximum noise level observed being more than

90 dB. Sources of noise in the OR are numerous and include the low humming of ventilation systems and other electronic equipment, alarms and feedback alerts on pumps and monitors, music, telephones ringing, pagers (beepers) sounding, people entering and existing the room, and sidebar conversations among surgical staff.[4,10] Noise can negatively affect surgical performance in a variety of ways, and these effects are particularly detrimental on dynamic tasks that require flexibility or rapid changes of responses to unexpected events. In particular, sources of noise can cause distraction and can hinder the ability of a surgeon to concentrate by masking acoustic task-related cues and inner speech so that surgeons cannot hear themselves think. Noise and distractions can also affect communication among the surgical team by reducing the ability to hear what others are saying or by causing statements spoken by others to be missed. Communication can also be hindered by changes in speech patterns that often occur when an individual needs to shout to overcome background noise.

Reducing noise and distractions in the OR is clearly desirable and would likely improve error management processes and surgical outcomes.[11,12] Policies that limit the number of observers in the operating theater, restrict the use of radios and pagers, curb nonessential staff from entering the OR during a case and discourage noncase-related conversations among the surgical team have all been recommended. Such policies may not be practical in all organizations or may not be readily accepted by surgical staff. For example, during long surgical cases, the presence of background music may help individuals maintain levels of mental arousal needed to combat the effects of fatigue or boredom. Furthermore, the ability to engage in noncase-related conversations among surgical staff might also contribute to team cohesion and job satisfaction. Likewise the inability to communicate with others outside the OR via telephone or pagers may affect the safety of other patients in the hospital who are also under the care of the surgeon (eg, in the postoperative intensive care unit) if alternative mechanisms or procedures for communication are not established. A compromise might be selective application of the sterile cockpit rule, limiting noise and distractions only during critical phases of an operation that imposes high mental workload, such as weaning the patient from the heart-lung machine. Among the challenges to application of this approach is the spectrum of tasks that impose high mental workload, which vary considerably across surgical staff as well as across different phases of the surgical procedure.[13,14]

TEAMWORK AND COMMUNICATION

Effective teamwork and communication have been recognized as imperative drivers of quality and safety in almost every complex industry. The Joint Commission (2006)[15] has identified communication as the number 1 root cause (65%) of reported sentinel events from 1995 to 2004. Within the surgical arena specifically, we have previously shown[4] that teamwork factors alone accounted for roughly 45% of the variance in the errors committed by surgeons during cardiac cases. Teamwork issues generally clustered around issues of miscommunication, lack of coordination, failures in monitoring, and lack of team familiarity. These findings are not specific to our study. Poor staff communication has been linked to poor surgical outcomes in general.[3,16] For example, a study by Gawande and colleagues[17] reported on the dangers of incomplete, nonexistent, or erroneous communication in the OR, indicating that such miscommunication events were causal factors in 43% of errors made during surgery. Another study by Lingard and colleagues[18] found that 36% of communication errors in the OR resulted in visible effects on system processes, including inefficiency, team tension, resource waste, work-around, delay, patient inconvenience, and procedural error.

A recent review of the teamwork literature[19] identified many team effectiveness models. Each of these models, in turn, highlights a variety of key factors that presumably promote better teamwork performance. However, the investigators concluded that there is currently no consensus among researchers as to how teamwork should be defined or the types of strategies that should be used to improve team effectiveness. Despite this situation, the empiric research on the breakdown of surgical teams' communication and coordination during cardiac surgery clearly indicated several possibilities for improving team performance, including strategies that focus on team training, standardized communication, team familiarity and stability, and preoperative briefings.[4] Although each has clear potential for enhancing safety, we focus on the last 2, because of their potentially unique fit with the surgical care process.

Cumulative Experience, Team Familiarity, and Stability

One of the key factors that affects teamwork and communication is team familiarity. For example, we recently compared miscommunication events during cardiac surgical cases among primary and secondary surgical teams.[20] Primary surgical teams were defined as those in which most team members (certified surgical technologist, circulating registered nurse, resident/fellow, perfusionist, certified registered nurse anesthetist/anesthesiologist) were routinely matched together during surgical cases, whereas secondary surgical teams consisted mostly of members who had little familiarity with the operating surgeon or other team members. Results revealed a significantly lower number of surgical flow disruptions including miscommunication events per case among familiar (primary) teams versus unfamiliar (secondary) surgical teams. An analysis of individual surgeon performance was also consistent with these findings, in that surgeons made significantly fewer surgical errors per case when working with their primary surgical teams than when working with secondary teams.

Carthey and colleagues[12] also found that team stability significantly improved the ability of cardiac surgeons to perform the complex aortic switch operation in pediatric patients. In particular, surgeons who had a different scrub nurse for each case, or worked in institutions that used ad hoc assignment of staff to the surgical theater, had more difficulty establishing team coordination at the table than surgeons who worked with familiar teams. During conditions in which surgeons were working with less familiar team members, they experienced "repeated losses of surgical flow because the team had to stop intermittently to correct errors." Similar observations have been made during cases in which changes of staff occur because of work breaks or shift turnover, which disrupts the continuity of the team and their shared knowledge of the events.

Team familiarity and stability can also improve process variables, in addition to reducing errors and patient safety issues. For example, surgical teams who attempted to adopt a new technology had significantly shorter operating times when original teams were kept intact. Furthermore, literature in both the medical and organizational fields has found team stability to be an independent predictor of team performance. Within the surgical arena, the cumulative experience of the team has also been shown to significantly decrease operative times, which may be secondary to fewer surgical flow disruptions because of miscommunication. In stable teams, trust develops amongst team members, which in turn produces psychological safety. Team stability also allows for the acquisition of familiarity of other team members' nonverbal communication styles and the anticipation of others' actions. In addition, as described in our previous study, stabilizing surgical teams would likely decrease staff turnover and increase team satisfaction.

It may be difficult within most institutions to allow only primary surgical team members to operate as a unit from a logistical standpoint; however, it is important that team members acquire an acceptable level of familiarity with one another. For example, at a minimum, one might strive for team stability during each surgical case. Team stability is important for developing and maintaining a shared mental model or awareness of the progression of the case, the potential problems that may have occurred previously during the case, or an understanding about any problems that may arise as the case progresses. One possible way of increasing team stability during an operation is to prohibit shift turnover (eg, the changing of surgical assistants or circulating nurses during a case), thereby requiring all surgical staff who began the case to remain in the OR until the operation is completed. However, such a strategy may be logistically implausible because of workload issues or professionally unacceptable given the culture within an organization (the topics of workload and organizational culture are discussed in depth in later sections). However, further research is clearly required to determine the effect that shift turnover might have on teamwork, as well as potential ways of remedying its impact.

Preoperative Briefings

Team meetings, such as preoperative briefings conducted before an operation, have the potential to address a variety of communication and teamwork issues. Preoperative briefings are not synonymous with the universal protocol or presurgical pause to ensure the right patient, right site, and right procedure. Briefings are meetings that are often conducted before the patient enters the OR and involve a more in-depth review of the case. Briefings also allow team members to ask questions or clarify uncertainties. Thus, preoperative briefings can be beneficial for all types of surgical teams, in terms of planning different aspects of the case, but may be principally beneficial for unfamiliar teams who may not be acquainted with a specific surgical procedure or the preferences of a particular surgeon. For example, DeFontes and Surbida[21] developed a preoperative briefing protocol for use by general surgical teams that was similar to a preflight briefing used by the airline industry. A 6-month pilot of the briefing protocol indicated that wrong-site surgeries decreased, employee satisfaction increased, nursing personnel turnover decreased, and perception of the safety climate in the OR improved from good to outstanding. Operating suite personnel's perception of teamwork quality also improved substantially. Within cardiac surgery, we found a significant reduction in the case frequency of surgical flow disruptions after implementation of preoperative briefings.[4] Specifically, there was a reduction in the number of procedural knowledge disruptions and miscommunication events per case. On average, teams that conducted the briefing had significantly fewer trips to the core and spent less time in the core during the surgical case. There was also a trend toward decreased waste for teams that were briefed compared with teams that did not conduct a preoperative briefing.

Despite the potential benefits of preoperative briefings, and the recent endorsement of briefings by the World Health Organization (2008),[22] their utilization remains low within many surgical specialties. This situation is likely a result of multiple factors. For example, there are no standardized protocols for conducting preoperative briefings. Each surgical specialty has unique issues that may need to be addressed before each operation. Therefore, a generic off-the-shelf checklist may not suffice. The development of a common template for designing briefing protocols is not unattainable, rather the specific content needs to be tailored to each surgical specialty. Other barriers impeding the use of preoperative briefings include individual attitudes or resistance to change by surgical staff, as well as organizational barriers such as case schedules, lack of facilities, and limited resources. As documented by DeFontes and Surbida,[21] the successful development of a preoperative briefing protocol takes several months of research and development, beginning with understanding the needs and views of key stakeholders (ie, surgical staff) and the nuances of the organization in which such briefings are to take place. There may also be confusion between 1-way communication via a checklist compared with bidirectional communication via an interactive and participatory briefing.

TOOLS AND TECHNOLOGY

The practice of surgery demands daily interface with highly sophisticated technologies. However, few of these medical technologies have been designed with the end user in mind, increasing the likelihood of user error.[21] However, poor design is not the only issue that can negatively affect performance and use of medical technology. The process by which new technology is introduced and implemented can also have an impact on user acceptance and use, affecting the delivery of safe and efficient surgical care. Even when technology is properly designed, its implementation can have unintended consequences on the work process, some of which may be inconsequential and others may be profound.

Ensuring that Technology is Usable and Acceptable

New technology is often difficult to use because it differs from its predecessors in terms of the method by which information is displayed, inputs are performed, and automation is provided.[23] Adjustment to new technology is even more difficult when systems are poorly designed. The role that poorly designed technology can play in producing errors that cause patient harm is becoming increasingly apparent. Roughly half of all recalls of medical devices result from design flaws, with specific types of devices being associated with unusually high use-error rates, such as infusion delivery devices. For example, in a previous human factor study of CPB machines, we identified several problems with the design and usability of these devices that predisposed surgical teams to make perfusion-related and other technical errors that threatened patient safety.[4] In particular, these design shortcomings included problems with the format, legibility, and integration of information across displays, the location, sensitivity, and shape of input controls, and problems with indistinguishable, unreliable, disarmed, or nonexistent audible alarms. Such problems have also often been cited as factors contributing to user error of medical devices in anesthesia and other health care settings.[24]

Research also suggests that health care providers are not passive recipients of new technology. Rather they are active agents who tailor technology to meet their needs, even if it is not effectively designed to do so. For example, Cook and Woods[23] studied cardiac anesthesiologists' use of a new computer-based physiology monitoring system during CPB procedures. Results revealed several characteristics of the new technology that reflected clumsy automation. Specifically, the benefits of the new computer system occurred during low workload situations but it also created new cognitive and physical demands that tended to congregate at times of high demand. As a result, anesthesiologists attempted to overcome these problems by adapting both the technology and their behavior to meet the needs of the patient during surgery, increasing the potential risk of errors. Other studies have found that users, rather than adapting to technology that is difficult to use, simply discontinue its use altogether.

Ensuring that medical devices and technology are designed to optimize their effective and safe use is clearly a priority in health care. The US Food and Drug Administration, US Department of Health and Human Services, and Center for Devices and Radiological Health jointly published the report *Medical Device Use Safety: Incorporating Human Factors Engineering into Risk Management*, which stated, "The field of human factors provides a variety of useful approaches to help identify, understand and address (medical device) use-related problems. The goal is to minimize use-related hazards, assure that intended users are able to use medical devices safely and effectively throughout the product life cycle." Performing usability testing and heuristic evaluations to ensure that medical devices meet minimal design standards is one basic approach for achieving this objective.[4] However, even when devices are deemed to be ergonomically designed, ensuring that end users have an opportunity to participate in the implementation process is vital to the acceptance of new technology. As noted by Lorenzi and Riley,[25] "a 'technically best' system can be brought to its knees by people who have low psychological ownership in the system and who vigorously resist its implementation." Training on the use of new technology is also important. For example, a recent study reported that surgeons are generally slower to adopt new information technology than their colleagues even when they believe it could potentially benefit patient care, because they often lack the appropriate training to use it effectively.[26] Although many of these issues regarding technology design and training are common knowledge to human factor engineers, challenges remain with regard to how to implement these best practices within the context of cardiac surgery.

Anticipating Unintended Consequences

New technology, even if well designed, can have complex effects on work systems and can fundamentally transform the nature of the work process in unforeseen ways and with unanticipated consequences.[23] The introduction of new surgical technology not only changes the nature of the task of the surgeon and the required psychomotor skills to accomplish it, it can also dramatically change the dynamics among the entire surgical team. For example, the introduction of minimally invasive cardiac surgery systems and surgical robots has been found to change the location of information sources, the information needs of surgeons, the nature of the visual information at the surgical site, and the flow of information exchange among the surgical staff.[27] Even changes to seemingly benign tools such as the whiteboard in the OR can have significant effects. A recent study examined the use of whiteboards and the potential impact that introducing electronic whiteboards might have on collaborative work within a trauma center operating suite.[28] Results suggested that the advantage of an electronic whiteboard with regard to automatic updating of information needed to be balanced against discouragement of active interaction and adaptation by surgical staff.[28] In particular, large electronic display boards do not necessarily replicate the social functions of the whiteboard, such as resource planning and tracking, synchronous and asynchronous communication, multidisciplinary problem solving and negotiation, and socialization and team building.

Clearly, the introduction of new technology can have unexpected interactions within the surgical team and can potentially induce new forms of error. New technology often requires adjustments in team communication, the development of new procedures, and altered roles of OR personnel.[27] Consequently, efforts need to be made before deployment to better understand how collaborative work may be affected in order to inform design and implementation strategies. Basic usability testing and heuristic evaluations can help in this process. However, simulation might serve as a more effective method for identifying unanticipated changes to work processes and it can also be useful for training in new procedures associated with adapting to the technology. Simulation should be designed into the implementation process because it provides a safe and efficient means of planning, training, and learning about how the introduction of the new technology changes the current work system and what changes need to be made to allow the new work system to function safely before the technology is adopted. However, not all organizations have the resources or facilities to conduct elaborate simulation evaluations, nor can simulations always adequately mimic the real-world scenarios surrounding the use of the technology in practice. Therefore, pilot testing of new technologies is also important because it allows for additional problems to be identified that may not have been discovered during usability or simulation testing. Nevertheless, the process of identifying unintended effects of new technology remains more of an art than science. Research is needed to develop and refine methods for reliably determining the impact of new technology before it is implemented.

TASK AND WORKLOAD FACTORS

Job task factors such as physical and mental workload can dramatically affect performance and safety.[27] Physical workload is often affected by task duration, strength requirements to complete the task, and behavioral repetition, whereas mental workload factors generally refer to the cognitive complexity (mental demand), time pressure, and criticality or risk of a task. Neither task dimension is completely independent of the other. Both types of workload can reduce levels of cognitive function by increasing levels of stress and fatigue, as is often the norm in complex high-intensity fields such as cardiac surgery.[29] As with most work system factors in the SEIPS model, several recommendations have been used in other industries for reducing both mental and physical workload, including the use of new technology (eg, automation) and the development of standardized procedures and checklists, as well as the incorporation of rest breaks into the work scheduling process. Issues related to the last 2 recommendations are discussed in the next section.

Developing Standardized Procedures and Checklists for Critical Tasks

Standardized procedures and checklists have long been used in other dynamic safety-critical environments such as aviation to decrease errors of omission (forgetting critical steps) and errors of commission (improper implementation of a procedure or protocol), and to reduce decision errors under stressful situations. In general, a checklist is "a list of action items, tasks or behaviors arranged in a consistent [standardized] manner, which allows the evaluator to record the presence or absence of the individual items listed."[29] As a result, the use of a checklist can be particularly beneficial when there is a long sequence of operations or multiple steps in a procedure, there are critical aspects or timing of a task that cannot be missed or forgotten, there are important or mandatory tasks that must be performed, or there are multiple tasks distributed across time or personnel. Under these conditions, the use of checklists and memory aids within critical care settings has been found to reduce errors and improve the quality and reliability of medical care through the use of best practices.[29] Checklists have also been shown to be beneficial and life saving in medical situations that require rapid systematic or standard approaches to crisis management such as anesthesiology[30] and emergency medicine.[31] Checklists are particularly useful when dealing with the human/machine interface.

Despite the proven benefits of checklists in improving the delivery of patient care, their integration into practice, including cardiac surgery, has not been so widespread as in other fields.[29] Perhaps one reason for this limited deployment of checklists is the concern that they reduce the flexibility of the health care provider. The implementation of a checklist might imply that it must be strictly adhered to in all situations, thereby potentially compromising the efficacy of the clinical process and infringing on clinical judgment.[29] The design of a checklist is also critical to its effectiveness. Poorly designed checklists can lead to errors and accidents, as has been shown in the aviation industry. There are no published data to indicate that checklists have contributed to adverse events in health care settings or delays in treatment because of length or poor design.[29]

Care also needs to taken when identifying which processes and procedures require the use of checklists so that they do not create an additional burden or layer of complexity.[4] As noted by Hales and colleagues,[29] "if each detail of every task were targeted for the development of a checklist, clinicians may experience 'checklist fatigue' whereby they become overburdened with completing these lists." Even when checklists are well designed, interruptions and distractions can still cause steps in a procedure to be missed or skipped. In addition, after several iterations of a procedure, complacency regarding task performance can arise, producing a perception that the checklist is unnecessary and therefore no longer used.[4] Consequently, users of checklists need to be trained in their use and committed to incorporating them into their practice. To achieve this goal, considerable human factor research is needed to understand the context and goals of checklist use, including the application of cognitive task analysis methods, as well as the inclusion of a multidisciplinary research team to ensure that checklists are properly designed and endorsed by users.

ORGANIZATIONAL INFLUENCES

Several organizational factors have the potential to affect the delivery of safe and reliable health care, and many of these factors have been discussed in the literature.[32] However, the topic of establishing and promoting a culture of safety within health care organizations "has become one of the pillars of the patient safety movement."[33] The general concept of a safety culture is not new and is generally traced back to the nuclear accident at Chernobyl in 1986, in which a poor safety culture was identified by the International Atomic Energy Agency as a major factor contributing to the accident. Since then, safety culture has been discussed in other major accident enquiries and analyses of system failures, such as the King's Cross Underground fire in London and the Piper Alpha oil platform explosion in the North Sea, as well as the crash of Continental Express Flight 2574, the Columbia Space Shuttle accident, and the explosion at the British Petroleum refinery in Texas City.

The concept of safety culture has also been applied to patient safety. Patient safety culture is defined as the enduring value and priority placed on patient care by everyone in every group at every level of a health care organization. It refers to the extent to which individuals and groups commit to personal responsibility for patient safety, act to preserve, enhance, and communicate patient safety concerns, strive to actively learn, adapt, and modify (both individual and organizational) behavior based on lessons learned from mistakes, and be rewarded in a manner consistent with these values. Although safety culture may not be the only determinant of safety in organizations, it plays a substantial role in encouraging people to behave safely and to report errors when they do occur. There is also growing evidence that interventions aimed at improving safety culture can reduce accidents and injuries[34] and within health care settings can reduce medical errors. Several strategies have been proposed for improving safety culture. However, as may be gleaned from its definition, the 2 interventions that seem to have the biggest potential are leadership engagement and accountability.

Improving Leadership Engagement

Leadership style has been shown to have a major impact on how patient safety initiatives are viewed and accepted among medical staff. Leaders who are considered engaging, transformational, and rewarding seem to have the most influence on improving safety culture. For example, Keroack and colleagues[32] found that chief executive officers (CEOs) at top performing institutions tended to be passionate about improving quality and safety, and tended to have a hands-on style. They were frequent visitors to patient care areas, either as part of structured leadership walk-rounds or as unscheduled observers. In contrast, CEOs at institutions that had struggling safety cultures were generally unsure of their leadership roles in quality and safety initiatives. In addition, staff reported rarely seeing them in care areas and indicated that they did not feel comfortable raising safety or quality concerns with CEOs directly. Others studies have also shown the benefits of improving leadership engagement through executive walk-rounds. For example, monthly executive walk-rounds have been shown to have a significant impact on improving safety culture among nurses in tertiary care hospitals.[35] Pronovost and colleagues[36] reported that improving leadership engagement in patient safety activities within an intensive care unit significantly improved safety culture, reduced length of stay, nearly eliminated medication errors in transfer orders, and decreased nursing turnover.

According to the Institute for Healthcare Improvement,[37] executive walk-rounds show a leader's commitment to safety and dedication to learn about the safety issues within their organizations. They also reflect an "organization's commitment to building a culture of safety." However, several issues need to be considered during the implementation of a walk-round strategy. For example, executives generally require training on how to conduct walk-rounds and how to ensure that walk-rounds remain informal. They also may need to be provided with tools or scripts to help them talk with front-line providers about safety issues and to show their support for staff-reported errors. In addition, some organizations are large and provide patient care around the clock, reducing the feasibility of having senior executives perform regular walk-rounds throughout all care units at different times of the day (or night). An alternative approach therefore has been to use an adopt-a-unit strategy, in which executives limit their walk-rounds to selected sites in a hospital rather than attempting to visit all units during a given period of time.[36]

Perhaps even more problematic is the process of attempting to conduct walk-rounds in surgical care units. In particular, a key component of walk-rounds that presumably makes them effective in changing culture is that leaders are seeking to actively engage front-line staff and providers in their own care setting. However, talking with cardiac surgeons, anesthesiologists, nurses, and perfusionists during bypass surgery would likely prove challenging. Consequently, executive walk-rounds with surgical staff may have to occur in the cafeteria or break room, or possibly in a town-hall setting such as during monthly staff meetings. However, whether such modifications to the walk-rounds strategy will prove to be equally effective in changing culture within a surgical care environment has yet to be determined.

The Role of the Surgeon

Within the current conceptualization of the SEIPS model, the central component around which all other OR work system factors revolve is the surgeon. However, the SEIPS model contrasts with traditional person-centered approaches that focus specifically on the negative consequences of surgical errors and disciplinary reactions to address them. Rather, the model focuses on factors that foster surgical excellence, as well as work system interventions to ensure that excellence is achieved and maintained. The SEIPS model clearly views the surgeon's cognitive flexibility, adaptability, and resiliency as being an important safety barrier between the work system factors in the OR and their potentially negative impact on patient safety. For example, Carthey and colleagues[11] found that surgeons who were able to cope with unexpected complications during surgery showed effective cognitive flexibility. Cognitive flexibility refers to the ability to consider multiple hypotheses when attempting to generate potential causes of a patient's unstable condition. Cognitive adaptability is also an important factor that can affect problem solving during surgical cases. For example, threats to patient safety decrease when surgeons are able to change their technique or strategy in light of unexpected patient anatomy, disruptions to surgical flow, or other unanticipated changes in work system events.[10]

When work system factors do disrupt surgical processes, a surgeon's mental resiliency is a key factor in ameliorating their impact on patient care. Mental resilience is reflected by the surgeon's ability to remain calm after ineffective attempts to remedy problems, as well as the capacity to maintain a belief throughout a problem that it is resolvable.[11] According to de Leval and colleagues,[16] a marker of surgical excellence is not error-free performance but rather the ability to manage errors and problems during an operation. Effective error management consists of several interdependent processes, including error recognition, error explanation, and error recovery. For example, in our previous study of cardiac surgeons, we found that surgeons made roughly 3.5 errors per hour; however, most of these errors were detected and remedied by the surgical team without any observable intraoperative impact on the patient.[4] Another study by Bann and colleagues[38] found that the ability of general surgeons to detect common surgical errors during a surgical skills training course significantly predicted their surgical performance on 2 subsequent surgical tasks (ie, cystectomy and enterotomy).

Surgeons can also play a vital role in buffering the impact that work system factors have on other members of the surgical team. For example, Carthey and colleagues[12] found that surgeons who were capable of adapting their surgical and communication style when operating with new or inexperienced team members were able to foster effective team coordination in a manner that reduced errors and improved patient outcomes. A study by Pisano and colleagues[39] identified several characteristics of cardiac surgical teams that predicted successful or unsuccessful adoption of new technology associated with minimally invasive cardiac surgery. Of primary importance was the surgeon's outlook toward the new technology. Those surgeons who actively encouraged team members, created an environment of psychological safety, and viewed the technology as a fundamental change in the way surgery is performed had greater success compared with those who viewed the technology as simply a plug-in program, making no effort to challenge the surgical team.

A surgeon's ability to manage errors or adapt to dynamic changes in work system variables is vital to ensuring patient safety. However, not all surgeons are equally adept or proficient in these areas. Some investigators have argued that these nontechnical abilities are generally intractable because they reflect the inherent skills and personalities of surgeons. On the contrary, at least 1 study suggests that these skills can be improved with the use of a well-designed training curriculum.[40] Surgeons are the final safety barrier between the work system factors in the OR and the potentially negative impact they might have on patient safety. Surgeons also play a pivotal role in ensuring that interventions to improve work system factors and reliability of cardiac surgical care are successful.

SUMMARY

In the past 50 years, significant improvements in surgical care have been achieved. Nevertheless, considerable variability in surgical outcomes still exists across institutions and individual surgeons; moreover, surgical errors that significantly affect patient safety continue to occur. Historically, surgical errors have been viewed as being determined primarily by the technical skill of the surgeon. However, focusing only on individual skill assumes that surgeons and other members of the surgical team perform highly and uniformly, regardless of the variable working conditions within the OR environment. Alternatively, a work systems approach recognizes that surgical skill alone is not sufficient to determine outcomes, because the process of delivering surgical care involves several interdependent variables, many of which vary across hospitals, ORs, or surgical cases, and most of which are not normally under the control of the surgical team. In this article, the SEIPS model is used to highlight the nature of many of these work system factors that affect surgical performance, including the OR environment, teamwork and communication, technology and equipment, tasks and workload factors, and organizational variables. If further improvements in the success rate and reliability of cardiac surgery are to be realized, interventions need to be developed to reduce the negative impact that work system failures can have on surgical performance. Some recommendations have been proposed here; however, several challenges remain.

REFERENCES

1. Vincent C, Moorthy K, Sarker SK, et al. Systems approaches to surgical quality and safety: from concept to measurement. Ann Surg 2004;239:475–82.
2. ElBardissi AW, Wiegmann DA, Dearani JA, et al. Application of the human factors analysis and classification system methodology to the cardiovascular surgery operating room. Ann Thorac Surg 2007;83:1412–8 [discussion: 8–9].
3. Carthey J, de Leval MR, Reason JT. The human factor in cardiac surgery: errors and near misses in a high technology medical domain. Ann Thorac Surg 2001;72: 300–5.
4. Wiegmann DA, ElBardissi AW, Dearani JA, et al. Disruptions in surgical flow and their relationship to surgical errors: an exploratory investigation. Surgery 2007; 142:658–65.
5. Healey AN, Primus CP, Koutantji M. Quantifying distraction and interruption in urological surgery. Qual Saf Health Care 2007;16:135–9.
6. Ofek E, Pizov R, Bitterman N. From a radial operating theatre to a self-contained operating table. Anaesthesia 2006;61:548–52.
7. Fanning J. Illumination in the operating room. Biomed Instrum Technol 2005;39: 361–2.
8. Brogmus G, Leone W, Butler L, et al. Best practices in OR suite layout and equipment choices to reduce slips, trips, and falls. AORN J 2007;86:384–94 [quiz: 95–8].
9. Ofek O, Karsak M, Leclerc N, et al. Peripheral cannabinoid receptor, CB2, regulates bone mass. Proc Natl Acad Sci U S A 2006;103:696–701.
10. Catchpole KR, Giddings AE, Wilkinson M, et al. Improving patient safety by identifying latent failures in successful operations. Surgery 2007;142:102–10.
11. Carthey J, Woodward S, Adams S, et al. Patient safety. Safe and sound. Health Serv J 2003;113(Suppl):2–6.
12. Carthey J. The role of structured observational research in health care. Qual Saf Health Care 2003;12(Suppl 2):ii13–6.

13. Wadhera RK, Parker SH, Burkhart HM, et al. Is the "sterile cockpit" concept applicable to cardiovascular surgery critical intervals or critical events? The impact of protocol-driven communication during cardiopulmonary bypass. J Thorac Cardiovasc Surg 2010;139:312–9.

14. Parker SE, Laviana AA, Wadhera RK, et al. Development and evaluation of an observational tool for assessing surgical flow disruptions and their impact on surgical performance. World J Surg 2010;34:353–61.

15. Joint Commission on Health Care Quality and Safety, 2006. Sentinel event statistics; 2006. Available at: http://www.jointcommission.org/SentinelEvents/Statistics/. Accessed November 18, 2011.

16. de Leval MR, Carthey J, Wright DJ, et al. Human factors and cardiac surgery: a multicenter study. J Thorac Cardiovasc Surg 2000;119:661–72.

17. Gawande AA, Studdert DM, Orav EJ, et al. Risk factors for retained instruments and sponges after surgery. N Engl J Med 2003;348:229–35.

18. Lingard L, Espin S, Whyte S, et al. Communication failures in the operating room: an observational classification of recurrent types and effects. Qual Saf Health Care 2004;13:330–4.

19. Salas E, Wilson KA, Burke CS, et al. Does crew resource management training work? An update, an extension, and some critical needs. Hum Factors 2006; 48:392–412.

20. ElBardissi AW, Wiegmann DA, Henrickson S, et al. Identifying methods to improve heart surgery: an operative approach and strategy for implementation on an organizational level. Eur J Cardiothorac Surg 2008;34:1027–33.

21. Defontes J, Surbida S. Preoperative safety briefing project. Permanente J 2004;8: 21–7.

22. World Health Organization's patient-safety checklist for surgery. Lancet 2008; 372(9632):1.

23. Cook RI, Woods DD. Adapting to new technology in the operating room. Hum Factors 1996;38:593–613.

24. Morrow D, North R, Wickens CD. Reducing and mitigating human error in medicine. Rev Hum Factors Ergon 2005;1:254–96.

25. Lorenzi NM, Riley RT. Managing change: an overview. J Am Med Inform Assoc 2000;7:116–24.

26. Lee MJ. Evidence-based surgery: creating the culture. Surg Clin N Am 2006;86: 91–100, ix.

27. Cao GL, Rogers G. Robotics in health care: HF issues in surgery. In: Carayon C, editor. Human factors and ergonomics in health care and patient safety. New Jersey: Lawrence Earlbaum; 2007. p. 411–21.

28. Xiao Y, Schenkel S, Faraj S, et al. What whiteboards in a trauma center operating suite can teach us about emergency department communication. Ann Emerg Med 2007;50:387–95.

29. Hales B, Terblanche M, Fowler R, et al. Development of medical checklists for improved quality of patient care. Int J Qual Health Care 2008;20:22–30.

30. Hart EM, Owen H. Errors and omissions in anesthesia: a pilot study using a pilot's checklist. Anesth Analg 2005;101:246–50, table of contents.

31. Harrahill M, Bartkus E. Preparing the trauma patient for transfer. J Emerg Nurs 1990;16:25–8.

32. Keroack MA, Youngberg BJ, Cerese JL, et al. Organizational factors associated with high performance in quality and safety in academic medical centers. Acad Med 2007;82:1178–86.

33. Nieva VF, Sorra J. Safety culture assessment: a tool for improving patient safety in healthcare organizations. Qual Saf Health Care 2003;12(Suppl 2):ii17–23.
34. Zohar D. Modifying supervisory practices to improve subunit safety: a leadership-based intervention model. J Appl Psychol 2002;87:156–63.
35. Thomas EJ, Sexton JB, Neilands TB, et al. Correction: the effect of executive walk rounds on nurse safety climate attitudes: a randomized trial of clinical units [ISRCTN85147255]. BMC Health Serv Res 2005;5:46.
36. Pronovost P, Weast B, Rosenstein B, et al. Implementing and validating a comprehensive unit-based safety program. J Patient Saf 2005;1:33–40.
37. Available at: http://www.ihi.org. Accessed December 15, 2010.
38. Bann S, Khan M, Datta V, et al. Surgical skill is predicted by the ability to detect errors. Am J Surg 2005;189:412–5.
39. Pisano GP, Bohmer RM, Edmondson AC. Organizational differences in rates of learning: evidence from the adoption of minimally invasive cardiac surgery. Manag Sci 2001;47:752–68.
40. Rogers AE, Hwang WT, Scott LD. The effects of work breaks on staff nurse performance. J Nurs Adm 2004;34:512–9.

Surgeons' Non-technical Skills

Steven Yule, MA, MSc, PhD, CPsychol[a,b,c],
Simon Paterson-Brown, MBBS, MPhil, MS, FRCS(Edin), FRCS(Engl), FCS(HK)[d],*

KEYWORDS

- Surgeons • Non-technical skills • Behavior rating
- Assessment

Over the last decade or so there has been increasing recognition that adverse events in health care, and specifically surgery, are more likely to originate from behavioral failures than a lack of technical expertise.[1,2] Analysis of worldwide literature suggests that as many as 10% to 15% of patients admitted to hospital experience an adverse event not directly related to their underlying condition, around 50% of which are classified as avoidable. Most of those patients are surgical,[3] and studies indicate that approximately half of all adverse events occur in the operating room (OR).[4] Much of the background information on these adverse events is covered elsewhere in this issue.

The recognition of the enormity of the scale of the problem worldwide led to the introduction of the World Health Organization (WHO) surgical checklist,[5] which showed a significant reduction in mortality and morbidity in a large multicountry study. A follow-up study performed in already high-performing hospitals in the Netherlands[6] confirmed the benefits of this checklist. However, data from the United States in relation to the persisting errors that still occurred after the adoption of the universal protocol[7] suggest that the checklist itself is not the panacea for avoiding adverse events, even if it does help to reduce them. This situation is undoubtedly because the checklist works, not just by providing a tick-box reminder of specific points but by having the underlying ability to focus the team on the job in hand and address some of the human factor issues around patient safety. If these issues are not understood then the full value of the checklist is lost.

These findings all support the argument that although technical skills are necessary for safe surgery, taken in isolation they are not sufficient to maintain high levels of performance over time. In addition, what are now commonly termed non-technical skills,[8] are as important, and sometimes more important, in ensuring the optimum outcome for the patient undergoing surgery. The problem within medicine in general,

---

[a] Department of Surgery, Harvard Medical School, 25 Shattuck Street, Boston, MA 02115, USA
[b] Director of Research and Education, STRATUS Center for Medical Simulation, Brigham & Women's Hospital, 75 Francis Street, Neville House, Boston, MA 02115, USA
[c] School of Psychology, University of Aberdeen, Regent Walk, Aberdeen, AB24 2UB, Scotland, UK
[d] Department of Clinical Surgery, Royal Infirmary, Little France, Edinburgh, EH16 4SA, Scotland, UK
* Corresponding author.
E-mail address: simon.paterson-brown@luht.scot.nhs.uk

Surg Clin N Am 92 (2012) 37–50
doi:10.1016/j.suc.2011.11.004   surgical.theclinics.com
0039-6109/12/$ – see front matter © 2012 Elsevier Inc. All rights reserved.

and surgery in particular, is that these non-technical skills have never been formally recognized, taught, or assessed. However, in the past decade several studies have revealed that surgeons believe that these skills are essential for safe performance and that they have also been found to be lacking in instances of adverse events for surgical patients. For example, in a reply to an anonymous postal survey, 68 consultant surgeons from all specialties in southeast Scotland identified 70 separate skills that they considered important in a successful surgical trainee.[9] Of these skills, only 19 (27%) were technical and 22 (31%) clinical, with 29 (41%) related to communication, teamwork, and application of knowledge. Communication was also identified as an important causal factor in 43% of errors made in surgery in a study performed in North America in 2003.[10] Other studies have indicated that teamwork[11] and decision making[12] have been lacking in instances of surgical failure.

Analysis of adverse events and accidents in other high-risk industries, such as civil aviation, offshore oil exploration, and nuclear power generation, have resulted in the development of training and assessment in non-technical skills. This training is more commonly called crew resource management training, for which behavior rating systems have been developed to assess these non-technical skills in a more formal manner in the workplace. One such example is the NOTECHS (Non-technical Skills for Pilots) system,[13] which comprises categories and elements of non-technical skills and is used to observe and rate pilots' behavior in the cockpit during both simulated and real flight. Although there is continuing debate about the relevance of adopting methods of aviation safety to improve health care safety,[14,15] the approach of developing specific behavior rating systems for use in the OR seems to be a sound one; several such systems now exist and these are discussed in the following section.

BEHAVIORAL MARKER SYSTEMS

Behavioral marker systems such as NOTECHS are methods to identify behaviors that contribute to superior or substandard performance based on a taxonomy of skills. A rating scale is also used in conjunction with the taxonomy. These marker systems are context-specific and must be developed for the situation in which they are to be used. For example, the NOTECHS system was developed and evaluated with subject matter experts from civil aviation.[16] If a high level of validity is required, it is no use taking behavior marker systems developed to assess pilots, scoring out "pilots", inserting "surgeons", and then expecting that these systems are appropriate to assess surgeons. For effective non-technical skills assessment, the system needs to be explicit, transparent, reliable, and valid for the domain in which it is being used.

Observational methods of improving safety in medicine were originally pioneered in anesthesia.[17] More recently, other observational studies have identified the individual, team, and organizational factors that seem to underlie surgical performance.[18–22] These observational systems have been used to drive development and adaption of behavioral rating tools in surgery such as:

1. OTAS (Objective Teamwork Assessment System)[23,24]: a teamwork assessment tool for 3 subteams based on a theoretic model of teamwork[25]
2. Oxford NOTECHS[26]: amended aviation tool for rating surgeons
3. Surgical NOTECHS[27]: amended aviation tool for rating surgical teams
4. NOTSS (Non-Technical Skills for Surgeons)[28]: de novo development with subject matter experts (surgeons) to observe and rate individual surgeons.

These tools all differ on how they were developed, for whom they were developed, the level of analysis used, and for what purpose. The following section describes the development of the NOTSS system, which was designed as an educational framework and is being used by surgeons and researchers in Europe, Australia, Japan, and North America.

THE NOTSS PROJECT

Just as the behavioral marker system for pilots[13] was systematically developed and subjected to experimental and practical evaluation for the aviation industry, a similar technique was used in the NOTSS project to develop a skills taxonomy for surgeons. The project was run by the University of Aberdeen, with a multidisciplinary steering group of surgeons, psychologists, and an anesthetist. The research drew on previous work in Scotland on surgical competence, professionalism, and the skills surgeons require to operate safely, and followed on from a similar project that developed a behavior rating system for anesthetists: the ANTS (Anaesthetists Non-Technical Skills) system.[29] The aim of the NOTSS project was to develop and test an educational system for assessment and training based on observed skills in the intraoperative phase of surgery. The system was developed from the bottom up with subject matter experts (attending surgeons), instead of adapting existing frameworks used in other industries. It was considered important to recognize and understand the unique aspects of non-technical skills in surgery and not to assume that those non-technical skills identified for pilots, nuclear power controllers, or anesthetists would be exactly mirrored in, or relevant to, surgery. An adapted model of systems design[30] was used to guide the iterative development of NOTSS through 3 phases of work from task analysis, through system design, to evaluation (**Fig. 1**). These phases related to the 3 objectives set by the NOTSS steering group in 2003:

1. To identify the relevant non-technical skills required by surgeons
2. To develop a system to allow surgeons to rate these skills, and
3. To test the system for reliability and usability.

Subject matter experts (consultant/attending surgeons) were involved at all stages of design and a steering group chaired by applied psychologists facilitated the process. This strategy ensured that the resulting system was designed by surgeons for surgeons and was written in surgical language, free of technical jargon and

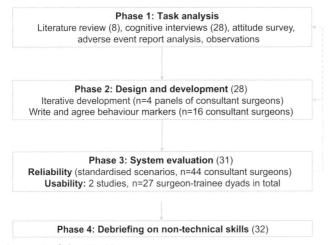

Phase 1: Task analysis
Literature review (8), cognitive interviews (28), attitude survey, adverse event report analysis, observations

Phase 2: Design and development (28)
Iterative development (n=4 panels of consultant surgeons)
Write and agree behaviour markers (n=16 consultant surgeons)

Phase 3: System evaluation (31)
Reliability (standardised scenarios, n=44 consultant surgeons)
Usability: 2 studies, n=27 surgeon-trainee dyads in total

Phase 4: Debriefing on non-technical skills (32)

Fig. 1. Development of the NOTSS system.

psychobabble. The resulting NOTSS taxonomy is broken down into 4 main categories, each with associated elements as shown in **Table 1**. The system is in surgical language for suitably trained surgeons to observe, rate, and provide feedback on non-technical skills in a structured manner. For each element, a judicious selection of good and poor behaviors was written; examples of these for situation awareness (SA) are shown in **Table 2**. This taxonomy was tested in a reliability study involving 44 consultant/attending surgeons, who were trained for 3 hours in the use of behavior markers and who then rated the lead surgeon's behaviors in a series of simulated operation scenarios. The social skills in NOTSS were found to be reliably rated across scenarios but the cognitive skill ratings were more variable.[31]

Subsequent phases of work have used the NOTSS system for debriefing trainees after surgery,[32] in surgical simulation, and as a central part of a master class to train surgeons to observe and rate non-technical skills.[33] NOTSS has also been subject to an independent trial of workplace assessment systems along with procedure-based assessment and OSATS (Objective Structured Assessment of Technical Skill),[34] with encouraging results in the OR[35]; it has been adopted by the Royal Australasian College of Surgeons as part of their competence assessment and is recommended by the Accreditation Council for General Medical Education.[36] A large-scale trial in Japanese hospitals is also under way.[37] A similar system has subsequently been developed for theater scrub practitioners (Surgical Practitioners' List of Intraoperative Non-Technical Skills [SPLINTS]).[38]

BREAKING DOWN NOTSS

The next sections discuss the 4 NOTSS categories (SA, decision making, communication and teamwork, and leadership), some of the problems associated with carrying them out correctly, and various solutions.

SA

Without good SA all the other non-technical skills struggle to succeed and it is worth taking time to establish exactly what is required for good SA, the problems in achieving it, and how these might be addressed. SA can be defined as developing and maintaining a dynamic awareness of the situation in the OR, based on assembling data from the environment (patient, team, time, displays, equipment); understanding

Table 1	
Non-technical skills taxonomy for surgeons	
Category	Element
Situation awareness	Gathering information
	Understanding information
	Projecting and anticipating future state
Decision making	Considering options
	Selecting and communicating option
	Implementing and reviewing decisions
Leadership	Setting and maintaining standards
	Supporting others
	Coping with pressure
Communication and teamwork	Exchanging information
	Establishing a shared understanding
	Coordinating team

Table 2
Examples of good and poor behaviors for situation awareness

Element	Good Behaviors	Poor Behaviors
Gathering information	Performs preoperative checks of patient notes Ensures that all relevant imaging/investigations have been reviewed and are available Liaises with anesthetist regarding anesthetic plan for patient Identifies anatomy/disease Monitors ongoing blood loss Asks anesthetist for update	Arrives in theater late or has to be called Does not ask for results until the last minute or not at all Does not consider the views of OR staff Fails to communicate with anesthetic team Asks anesthetist to read from patient notes during procedure because not read before operation started Fails to review information collected by team
Understanding information	Changes surgical plan in light of changes in patient condition Acts according to information gathered from previous investigation Looks at computed tomography (CT) scan and points out relevant area Reflects and discusses significance of information with team Communicates priorities to team	Overlooks or ignores important results Asks questions that show lack of understanding Poorly coordinates investigation Misses clear sign on CT scan Discards results that don't fit the picture
Projecting and anticipating future state	Shows evidence of having a contingency plan (plan B) by asking scrub nurse for potentially required equipment to be available in theater Keeps anesthetist informed about procedure (eg, to expect bleeding) Verbalizes what may be required later in operation Cites contemporary literature on anticipated clinical event	Overconfident maneuvers with no regard for what may go wrong Does not discuss potential problems with team Gets into predictable blood loss, then tells anesthetist Waits for a predicted problem to arise before responding

what they mean, and thinking ahead about what may happen next. According to Endsley's model,[39] SA comprises 3 distinct elements (levels): level 1 (gathering information); level 2 (interpreting the information) (and experience clearly plays a role here); and level 3 (projecting and anticipating future states based on this information).

Level 1
Information coming in (to the surgeon) does so from several sources, including the patient (anatomy), colleagues (verbal cues), and instruments (patient monitors). The OR is a busy and sometimes noisy place and a great deal of activity goes on (**Fig. 2**). It is therefore common for the surgeon to be concentrating so intensely on what they are doing that information is either not seen or not heard, or the importance not recognized (**Fig. 3**). This situation is what is often called inattentional blindness[40] or tunnel vision. This observation is not to say that the surgeon should not be concentrating hard on a specific task, but, by doing so, important information on the state of the patient or environment might go unrecognized and this should be realized.

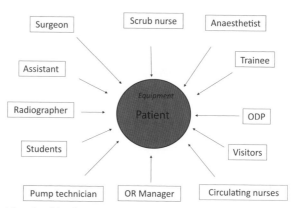

Fig. 2. Personnel involved in the OR.

Messages may need to be repeated and confirmed, background music may need to be turned off, and when things do get difficult and fraught, the principle of the sterile cockpit could be considered.[41] This strategy, not surprisingly, comes from aviation, when, usually during takeoff and landing (eg, less than 1524 meters [5000 ft]), no nonessential conversation should take place, thereby allowing the pilots to concentrate on the job in hand. Depending on the situation, the surgeon may ask for information to be repeated, request opinions from colleagues, or backtrack and go over previous information again to double-check comprehension.

Level 2
The surgeon needs to not only receive all the information but also to understand its significance. This ability requires a degree of training and experience, so junior surgeons, not aware of the significance of certain facts, respond (or do not respond) differently from senior, more experienced surgeons. A common problem in correctly

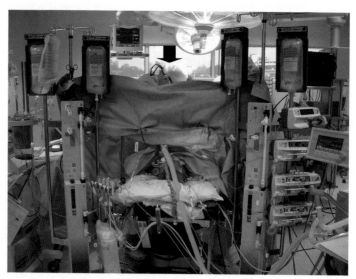

Fig. 3. Activities around the surgeon.

interpreting the information is confirmation bias. Information coming in is filtered to allow the surgeon to confirm their views, discarding any information that might suggest another cause. This situation can be avoided by analyzing all the information that comes in, and if necessary, discussing the potential diagnoses with other members of the team. A common reason for ignoring some information and accepting others may be that the alternative diagnosis suggests a radical change of plan that may be difficult or unpleasant.

Level 3

Having received and (it is hoped) recognized the importance of the information, the surgeon must then anticipate potential future events. This situation may or may not require a change of plan. Problems with incorrect anticipation may be avoided by discussing options with colleagues and reviewing alternatives.

This is all a dynamic situation and changes as the operation progresses. Surgeons with good SA regularly step back (to avoid tunnel vision) and reassess the situation, take on board all the relevant information including nonverbal clues (anesthetic activity, scrub nurse anxiety, and monitor warnings), and reconsider the operative plan based on revised assessment.

Decision Making

Decision making can be defined as skills for coming to a particular course of action.[42] There is now increasing interest in intraoperative judgment.[43] Classic models of decision making propose that this is an analytical process: the relative features of options are compared in turn and an optimal course of action is selected; for example; in cases of large bowel obstruction the surgeon might weigh up the various pros and cons of performing a primary anastomosis against a colostomy. Decision making can be an effortful process and requires both experience and time to come to an acceptable solution. It seems that during the intraoperative phase of surgery, surgeons use analytical decision making in around 50% of cases.[44]

Another common method of decision making applicable to intraoperative surgery is rule-based decision making. This method is used by trainee and expert surgeons alike and follows the "if X then Y" process. This process makes decision making easier, because once a situation has been detected, a relevant rule can be applied, either by consulting a manual or by referring to national guidelines or local protocols. Less formally, surgeons may remember anecdotal rules learnt during training that can be applied when certain situations arise. Deciding when to use antibiotic prophylaxis during surgery to reduce the risk of surgical site infection is 1 example.

However, experts tend to use a more heuristic-based style called recognition-primed decision making (RPD). This is a type of pattern matching that experts can use to make satisfactory decisions under times of high stress or time pressure. Studies on fire ground commanders and military decision makers[45] found that experts could often identify the first workable solution to a problem based on their experience rather than going through the effortful process of systematically generating options and comparing the features of those options before arriving at an optimal solution. The mental efficiency that RPD brings is important, because working memory space is diminished during times of acute stress. When a trainee surgeon seems to freeze at the operating table when faced with a difficult and stressful situation, this is probably because they have inadequate working memory for analytical decision making and do not have the experience to use RPD. The causes and effects of stress are discussed later in this article.

The final method is creative decision making, which, although sounding innovative, is usually only a last resort when the other methods are not possible or have been tried and found to be unsuccessful. Making such creative decisions can sometimes be successful but usually results in failure.

Communication and Teamwork

Communication and teamwork can be defined as the skills required for working in a team context to ensure that the team has an acceptable shared picture of the situation and can complete tasks effectively. What is essential is that each member of the team has a shared mental model of both what is happening and what is the planned outcome (**Fig. 4**). There are many barriers to communication, both internal and external, and these are summarized in **Box 1**.

Several studies have shown that many of the adverse events that occur in surgery relate to problems with communication[10–12] and these communication failures systematically recur.[46] Several general remedies for improving communication within the team have been developed and are summarized in **Table 3**.

When communication is improved, the shared mental model is undoubtedly better and teamwork benefits. Various tools have been developed to improve and clarify communication. CUSS is one in which assertive communication uses the following escalation[47]:

C "I'm concerned and need clarification"
U "I am uncomfortable and don't understand"
S "I'm seriously worried here"
S "stop"

Alternatively the ISBAR system, devised by the American military for precise and succinct transmission of messages, can be used[48]:

I Identify: who, where?
S Situation: what is the problem?
B Background: relevant PMH, presentation
A Assessment: what do you make of the problem?
R Recommendation: what do you think you should do?

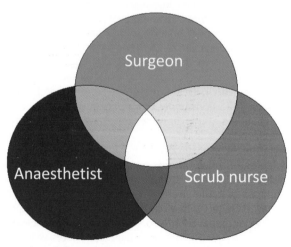

Fig. 4. Shared mental model.

Box 1
Barriers to communication
Internal
• Language difference
• Culture
• Motivation
• Expectations
• Past experience
• Status
• Emotions/mood
External
• Noise
• Low voice
• Deafness
• Electrical interference
• Separation in space and time
• Lack of visual cues (eg, body language, eye contact, gestures, facial expressions)

Use of these systems in isolation or by only selected members of the team does not lead to any real improvement in communication.

Leadership

There is widespread recognition in organizations exposed to hazards that leadership is essential for efficient and safe team performance. In the cognitive interviews as part of phase 1 of NOTSS development,[28] surgeons either described leadership in the OR as entirely their own responsibility, or as a shared responsibility between the surgeon, anesthetist, and nursing team leader. During the NOTSS development process, the leadership behaviors were grouped into 3 elements: setting and maintaining standards, supporting others, and coping with pressure. These social leadership skills were more reliably rated than cognitive skills in NOTSS.[49] However, according to a recent review of the literature,[50] there is limited empiric evidence identifying specific

Table 3	
Strategies for improving communication	
Problem	**Solution**
Misunderstanding information	Do not make assumptions
Information confusing	Be precise and clear
Information not heard/message ambiguous	Acknowledge receipt of information; verify information received; clarify any possible ambiguity
Sender uses hint-and-hope strategy	Say what you mean
Information given too early/too late	Pick your moment (especially if things are fraught)

leadership skills and associated behaviors enacted by surgeons during operations. Despite this paucity of research, some emerging studies have shown observations about surgeons' leadership behaviors that do not necessarily fit with traditional models from the leadership literature. In 1 recent observational study of 29 operations[51] a total of 258 surgical leadership behaviors were classified. The operating surgeons most frequently showed leadership behaviors classified as guiding and supporting (33%), communicating and coordinating (20%), and task management (15%). In many instances surgeons' leadership communications were not specifically directed to a particular team member. Accounting for operation length, surgeons engaged in leadership behaviors significantly more frequently during cases of high complexity compared with cases of lower complexity.[52] Other research on surgeons' intraoperative leadership suggests that residents move from emphasizing transactional to transformational behaviors as they progress through their training.[53]

The Surgical Checklist and NOTSS

As mentioned earlier, to provide a final error trap before surgery, the WHO "Safer Surgery Saves Life" campaign introduced the concept of the surgical checklist and the surgical pause (http://www.who.int/features/factfiles/safe_surgery/en). In addition to providing a final check before surgery, it has undoubtedly contributed to improving the various non-technical skills required for better operative surgery. SA around the diagnosis and procedure, along with the instruments/equipment required and possible difficulties that may be encountered (projection/anticipation), are all discussed. Decision making is improved by early identification of possible difficulties, and communication throughout the team is expressed audibly and acknowledged. Teamwork has to be improved by the knowledge of all the names of people in the OR, something that has often been neglected in the past, with many OR personnel not being known by name to each other, especially across specialties. Good leadership can be encouraged, and developed, by completing the checklist in the appropriate manner, showing a commitment to patient safety and both recognizing the roles and supporting other members of the operating team.

Stress and Fatigue

Although fatigue and stress are not non-technical skills, it is important to recognize how they can influence non-technical skills and how their effects can be mitigated against and managed to improve performance.

Stress

There has been increasing focus on the negative effects of stress (defined as when the demands on an individual outweigh the amount of control they are able to exert) and burnout in surgery. This focus has been partly because of the recently reported results of a large survey of 7905 surgeons in the United States that reported that more than 40% felt burned out,[54] a psychological term for chronic emotional exhaustion and diminished interest: a state that affects performance at work and can make surgical care less safe for patients. Burnout is one of the most serious outcomes of chronic stress, but the effects of stress manifest themselves in many other discrete and subtle ways. A systematic review of the literature on acute stress in surgery[55] found 22 empiric papers in a disparate field with a mix of subjective (eg, questionnaire) and objective (eg, heart rate, salivary cortisol) measurements of stress that were used by researchers working in the real OR as well as simulated settings. This review reported that the main stressors were the act of surgery itself; patient factors such as unanticipated bleeding; and noise, visitors, and distractions. Laparoscopic surgery was found to be more stressful than open surgery. Stress has been shown to affect technical as well as non-technical performance and although no controlled studies have been conducted in this area, experienced surgeons not surprisingly seem to be able to cope with stress better than juniors. Of particular importance are the changes in cognitive function associated with acute stress that significantly reduce available working memory and therefore have a detrimental effect on perception, decision making, and task management. As a result, decision making in acutely stressful situations may rely entirely on the RPD model; if someone lacks the experience for this, they may freeze and be unable to make a decision.

Fatigue

Fatigue is a factor in most commonly occurring accidents, including road traffic accidents and accidents in health care and other high-risk industries. Fatigue can be defined as a state of sleepiness characterized by feeling drowsy or tired that results in a reduced ability to maintain concentration, make decisions, and carry out skilled tasks. Lack of sleep is the most common cause of fatigue; sufferers are unable to think clearly and imaginatively, are more rigid in their thinking, and accept lower standards of performance. Motor skills are degraded and fatigued individuals are more prepared to accept their own errors, to become irritable and distracted, and are less tolerant of others. Moderate sleep loss is equivalent to moderate alcohol consumption in the way that it degrades motor performance.[56,57] It has now also been shown that decreasing hours of work for doctors reduces error.[58] Sleep is the only effective way of recovering from fatigue; after a short period of sleep deprivation it is possible to return to normal with 1 or 2 nights of good-quality sleep. It is well known that shift work disrupts normal sleep patterns by interrupting the circadian rhythm of the body and disrupting sleep cycles; however, working a single or a few night shifts can be recovered from quickly.[59,60] A week of nights is probably the worst pattern of work because fatigue accumulates toward the end of the week with disrupted sleep. Increasing age is associated with longer recovery time from periods of disturbed or reduced sleep, providing more justification for the more senior surgeons to come off the on-call rota.

SUMMARY

The appreciation of the importance of non-technical skills to surgical performance is now gaining wider acceptance. This article describes the core cognitive and social skill categories in this area. Several tools have been developed to rate these non-technical skills in the OR, focusing on observational methods as a means of assessment. These tools are being used informally by research groups and interested clinicians, but if the increase of non-technical skills appreciation in surgery mirrors that in other high-risk industries, such as civil aviation and nuclear power generation, these skills may need to be taught and assessed in a formative manner on a larger scale. The different taxonomies developed for use in the OR differ slightly in the balance of skill categories believed to be important. There are minor differences between the varieties of NOTECHS and NOTSS, but there are larger differences in the taxonomies developed for different clinical groups in the OR. For example, the skills identified in the NOTSS taxonomy are different from the taxonomies developed for both anesthetists and scrub practitioners because each taxonomy reflects the particular role of that profession within the operating team. In the ANTS taxonomy, task management was included as a category whereas leadership (included in NOTSS) was not. The prototype SPLINTS taxonomy contains only 3 categories because that was the number of high-level themes that emerged from task analysis in that domain.[61]

More work is needed in this area of surgery, but at present we know that good surgeons usually have good non-technical skills and most adverse events in surgery relate to poor non-technical skills. Furthermore, we now understand and recognize these non-technical skills. The challenge in the future is to incorporate them into undergraduate teaching, postgraduate training, assessment, and perhaps even selection.

REFERENCES

1. Bogner M, editor. Human error in medicine. Hillsdale (NJ): Lawrence Erlbaum Associates; 1994.
2. Bogner M, editor. Misadventures in health care. Mahwah (NJ): Lawrence Erlbaum Associates; 2004.
3. Vincent C, Neale G, Woloshynowych M. Adverse events in British hospitals: preliminary retrospective record review. BMJ 2001;322:517–9.
4. Flin R, Mitchell L. Safer surgery: analysing behaviour in the operating theatre. Aldershot (United Kingdom): Ashgate; 2009.
5. Haynes AB, Weiser TG, Berry WR, et al. A surgical safety checklist to reduce morbidity and mortality in a global population. N Engl J Med 2009;360:491–9.
6. Devries EN, Prins HA, Crolla RM, et al. Effect of a comprehensive surgical safety system on patient outcomes. N Engl J Med 2010;363:1928–37.
7. Stahel P, Sabel AL, Victoroff MS, et al. Wrong-site and wrong-patient procedures in the universal protocol era (analysis of a prospective database of physician self-reported occurrences). Arch Surg 2010;145:978–84.
8. Yule S, Flin R, Paterson-Brown S, et al. Non-technical skills for surgeons: a review of the literature. Surgery 2006;139:140–9.
9. Baldwin PJ, Paisley AM, Paterson-Brown S. Consultant surgeons' opinions of the skills required of basic surgical trainees. Br J Surg 1999;86:1078–82.
10. Gawande AA, Zinner MJ, Studdert DM, et al. Analysis of errors reported by surgeons at three teaching hospitals. Surgery 2003;133:614–21.
11. Christian CK, Gustafson ML, Roth EM, et al. A prospective study of patient safety in the operating room. Surgery 2006;139:159–76.
12. Greenberg CC, Regenbogen SE, Studdert DM. Patterns of communication breakdowns resulting in injury to patients. J Am Coll Surg 2007;204:533–40.
13. Flin R, Martin L. Behavioural marker systems in aviation. Int J Aviat Psychol 2001; 11:95–118.
14. Gaba D. Have we gone too far in translating ideas from aviation to patient safety? No. BMJ 2011;342:c7310.
15. Rogers J. Have we gone too far in translating ideas from aviation to patient safety? Yes. BMJ 2011;342:c7309.
16. Flin R, Martin L, Goeters K, et al. The development of the NOTECHS system for evaluating pilots' CRM skills. Hum Factors Aero Saf 2003;3:95–117.
17. Fletcher GC, McGeorge P, Flin RH, et al. The role of non-technical skills in anaesthesia: a review of current literature. Br J Anaesth 2002;88:418–29.
18. Helmreich RL, Davies JM. Human factors in the operating room: interpersonal determinants of safety, efficiency and morale. Baillieres Clin Anaesthesiol 1996; 10:277–95.
19. de Leval MR, Carthey J, Wright DJ, et al. Human factors and cardiac surgery: a multicentre study. J Thorac Cardiovasc Surg 2000;119(4):661–72.
20. Carthey J, de Leval MR, Reason JT. The human factor in cardiac surgery: errors and near misses in a high technology medical domain. Ann Thorac Surg 2001;72:300–5.

21. Fin R, O'Conner P, Crichton M. Safety at the sharp end. Aldershot (United Kingdom): Ashgate; 2008.
22. Catchpole KR, Giddings AE, Wilkinson M, et al. Improving patient safety by identifying latent failures in successful operations. Surgery 2007;142:102–10.
23. Healy AN, Undre S, Vincent CA. Developing observational measures of performance in surgical teams. Qual Saf Health Care 2004;13(Suppl 1):i33–40.
24. Undre S, Sevdalis N, Healey AN, et al. The Observational Teamwork Assessment for Surgery (OTAS): refinement and application in urological surgery. World J Surg 2007;31:1373–81.
25. Dickinson TL, McIntyre RM. A conceptual framework for teamwork measurement. In: Brannick MT, Salas E, Prince C, editors. Team performance assessment and measurement: theory, methods, and applications. Series in applied psychology. Mahwah (NJ): Lawrence Erlbaum Associates; 1997. p. 19–43.
26. Mishra A, Catchpole K, McCulloch P. The Oxford NOTECHS system: reliability and validity of a tool for measuring teamwork behaviour in the operating theatre. Qual Saf Health Care 2009;18:104–8.
27. Sevdalis N, Lyons M, Healey AN, et al. Observational teamwork assessment for surgery: construct validation with expert versus novice raters. Ann Surg 2009; 249:1047–51.
28. Yule S, Flin R, Paterson-Brown S, et al. Development of a rating system for surgeons' non-technical skills. Med Educ 2006;40:1098–104.
29. Fletcher G, Flin R, McGeorge P, et al. Anaesthetists' Non-Technical Skills (ANTS): evaluation of a behavioural marker system. Br J Anaesth 2003;90:580–8.
30. Gordon SE. Systematic training programme design: maximising effectiveness and minimizing liability. Englewood Cliffs (NJ): Prentice Hall; 1993.
31. Yule S, Flin R, Maran N, et al. Surgeons' non-technical skills in the operating room: reliability testing of the NOTSS behaviour rating system. World J Surg 2006;32:548–56.
32. Yule S, Flin R, Rowley D, et al. Debriefing surgical trainees on non-technical skills (NOTSS). Cognit Techn Work 2008;10:265–74.
33. Royal College of Surgeons of Edinburgh–see 'courses' Available at: http://www.rcsed.ac.uk/. Accessed July 27, 2011.
34. Martin JA, Regehr G, Reznick R, et al. Objective structured assessment of technical skill (OSATS) for surgical residents. Br J Surg 1997;84:273–8.
35. Crossley J, Marriott J, Purdie H, et al. Prospective observational study to evaluate NOTSS (Non-Technical Skills for Surgeons) for assessing trainees' non-technical performance in the operating theatre. Br J Surg 2011;98:1010–20.
36. Swing SR, Clyman SG, Holmboe ES, et al. Advancing resident assessment in graduate medical education. J Grad Med Educ 2009;1(2):278–86.
37. Yule S, Wilkinson G. Test of cultures. Surgeons News. October 2009. Available at: http://tinyurl.com/cdesyhr. Accessed November 18, 2011.
38. Mitchell L, Flin R. Non-technical skills of the operating theatre scrub nurse: literature review. J Adv Nurs 2008;61:15–24.
39. Endsley M, Garland D. Situation awareness. Analysis and measurement. Mahwah (NJ): Lawrence Erlbaum Associates; 2000.
40. Simons DJ, Chabris CF. Gorillas in our midst: sustained inattentional blindness for dynamic events. Perception 1999;28:1059–74.
41. Wadhera R, Henrickson Parker S, Burkhart H, et al. Is the "sterile cockpit" concept applicable to cardiovascular surgery critical intervals or critical events? The impact of protocol-driven communication during cardiopulmonary bypass. J Thorac Cardiovasc Surg 2010;139:312–9.

42. Flin R, Youngson GG, Yule S. How do surgeons make intraoperative decisions? Qual Saf Health Care 2007;16:235–9.
43. Jacklin R, Sevdalis N, Harries C, et al. Judgment analysis: a method for quantitative evaluation of trainee surgeons' judgments of surgical risk. Am J Surg 2008; 195:183–8.
44. Pauley K, Flin R, Yule S, et al. Surgeons' intra-operative decision making and risk management. Am J Surg 2011;202(4):375–81.
45. Klein G. A recognition-primed decision (RPD) model of rapid decision making. In: Klein G, Orasanu J, Calderwood R, et al, editors. Decision making in action. New York: Ablex; 1993. p. 138–47.
46. Lingard L, Espin S, Whyte S, et al. Communication failures in the operating room: an observational classification of recurrent types and effects. Qual Saf Health Care 2004;13:330–4.
47. Clarke J. Is my patient safe in the operating room? 2007. Available at: http://www.health.state.ny.us/professionals/patients/patient_safety/conference/2007/docs/is_my_patient_safe_in_the_operating_room.pdf. Accessed July 27, 2011.
48. Haig KM, Sutton S, Whittington J. SBAR: a shared mental model for improving communication between clinicians. Jt Comm J Qual Patient Saf 2006;32:167–75.
49. Yule S, Rowley D, Flin R, et al. Experience matters: comparing novice and expert ratings of non-technical skills using the NOTSS system. ANZ J Surg 2009;79: 154–60.
50. Henrickson Parker S, Yule S, Flin R, et al. Towards a model of surgeons' leadership in the operating room. BMJ Qual Saf 2011;20(7):570–9.
51. Henrickson Parker S, Yule S, Flin R, et al. Surgeons' leadership in the operating room: an observational study. Am J Surg, in press.
52. Edmondson A. Speaking up in the operating room: how team leaders promote learning in interdisciplinary action teams. J Manag Stud 2003;40:1419–52.
53. Horowitz IB, Horowitz SK, Daram P, et al. Transformational, transactional, and passive-avoidant leadership characteristics of a surgical resident cohort: analysis using the multifactor leadership questionnaire and implications for improving surgical education curriculums. J Surg Res 2008;148:49–59.
54. Shanaflet TD, Balch CM, Bechamps GJ, et al. Burnout and career satisfaction among American surgeons. Ann Surg 2009;250:463–71.
55. Arora S, Sevdalis N, Nestel D, et al. The impact of stress on surgical performance: a systematic review of the literature. Surgery 2010;147:318–30.
56. Williamson AM, Feyer AM. Moderate sleep deprivation produces impairments in cognitive and motor performance equivalent to legally prescribed levels of alcohol intoxication. Occup Environ Med 2000;57(10):649–55.
57. Roehrs T, Burduvali E, Bonahoom A, et al. Ethanol and sleep loss: a 'dose' comparison of impairing effects. Sleep 2003;26:981–5.
58. Lockley SW, Cronin JW, Evans EE, et al, Harvard Work Hours, Health and Safety Group. Effect of reducing interns' weekly work hours on sleep and attentional failures. N Engl J Med 2004;351(18):1829–37.
59. Wedderburn A. Guidelines for shiftworkers. Bulletin of European shiftwork topics, no. 3. Dublin (Ireland): European Foundation for the Improvement of Living and Working Conditions; 1991.
60. Spencer MB, Robertson KA, Folkard S. The development of a fatigue/risk index for shiftworkers. London: HSE Books; 2006.
61. Mitchell L, Flin R, Yule S, et al. Thinking ahead of the surgeon–an interview study to identify scrub practitioners' non-technical skills. Int J Nurs Stud 2011;48: 818–28.

A Comprehensive Unit-Based Safety Program (CUSP) in Surgery: Improving Quality Through Transparency

Michol Cooper, MD, PhD[a], Martin A. Makary, MD, MPH[b],*

KEYWORDS

- Wrong site • Wrong patient • Universal protocols
- Transparency

THE SCIENCE FOR COMPREHENSIVE UNIT-BASED SAFETY PROGRAM (CUSP) IN SURGERY

Medical care is expanding in a way that is becoming more fragmented, making opportunities for medical errors more common. Patients are increasingly falling through the cracks or being harmed by confusion among providers. Sometimes a process of care is too complex to be safe. Other times mistakes happen because of a simple lack of communication. These problems require common-sense solutions, many times necessitating changes to the way care is delivered on a local level. Specifically, unit-based meetings to discuss how local systems are potentially dangerous for patients are needed to streamline care and eliminate safety hazards. These comprehensive safety programs unite physicians, nurses, technicians, and other staff in a regular meeting to take on individual safety hazards identified by each group. After all, who knows what's best for a patient more than the doctors, nurses, and other team members that care directly for them? The implementation of a safety program typically includes the measurement of the unit's safety culture and inclusion of hospital management. Representation from management allows for resources to be allocated more efficiently, and also serves to bridge the growing

Financial disclosures: The authors have nothing to disclose.

[a] Department of Surgery Johns Hopkins Hospital, 600 North Wolfe Street, Baltimore, MD 21231, USA

[b] Department of Surgery, Johns Hopkins Hospital, Osler 624, 600 North Wolfe Street, Baltimore, MD 21231, USA

* Corresponding author.

E-mail address: mmakary1@jhmi.edu

Surg Clin N Am 92 (2012) 51–63
doi:10.1016/j.suc.2011.11.008
0039-6109/12/$ – see front matter © 2012 Elsevier Inc. All rights reserved.

surgical.theclinics.com

divide between hospital administration and front-line providers. Surgery unit safety programs draw on many lessons learned in the literature and explored in this article, and they also serve to customize safety interventions (eg, the surgical checklist) using local wisdom.

In recent years, there has been an increased focus on the causes and prevention of medical errors, particularly in surgery. Medical errors can cause catastrophic injuries to patients and can have significant consequences for the surgeon and institution. Although mistakes are inherent in human nature, many mistakes can be attributed to large and vulnerable health care systems.

In 1999, the Institute of Medicine (IOM) published one of the first and most important documents raising awareness of injuries due to medical errors, *To Err is Human: Building a Safer Health System*.[1] This report concluded that in American hospitals between 44,000 and 98,000 deaths and 1 million injuries occur each year due to medical error, amounting to more deaths in hospitals from medical errors than from motor vehicle accidents, breast cancer, and AIDS combined.[1] The report shocked the medical community, and after its publication talking about mistakes became more acceptable. Over time, professional associations and medical centers began having honest conversations about how systems can be more safely engineered so that mistakes can be prevented. To this end, over the last decade hospitals have embarked on many quality improvement campaigns. However, despite this a retrospective study of 10 hospitals in North Carolina followed for patient harm from 2002 to 2007 showed that 25.1% of all inpatients had sustained a form of preventable harm due to a medical mistake.[2] This finding shows that despite much attention in the medical community to improving patient safety and despite implementation of broad-sweeping quality measures, the field is still in its infancy. However, studies using sound scientific methods are beginning to populate the surgical literature.

NEVER EVENTS

In the nomenclature for quality and safety in health care, never events have become the most universally recognized quality indicator in surgery. Although the surgical community may disagree about quality metrics in general, there is universal agreement that never events represent preventable harm. Never events include wrong-site/wrong-patient surgery, an unintentional retained foreign body, and unexpected intraoperative death in a patient of American Society of Anesthesiologists (ASA) class I.[3] Never events have become a quality measure that is now closely monitored, although hospitals are not currently transparent with the public about how many of these events occur each year. Increasingly there is a trend to request that hospitals publicly report their rates of never events yearly.

WRONG-SITE/WRONG-PATIENT SURGERY

One of the most devastating medical errors to both patient and physician is wrong-site or wrong-patient surgery. Wrong-site surgery is defined as any surgical procedure performed on the wrong patient, wrong side of the body, wrong body part, or the wrong level of a correctly identified anatomic site. Wrong-patient surgery may include patients who were never scheduled for a procedure, procedures that were performed but were never scheduled, and procedures that were scheduled correctly but were never performed.[4] In the past these errors were believed to be extremely rare.[5] However, the incidence of these events ranges from 1 in 112,994 to up to 1 in 15,500 cases, and they can have disastrous health and financial consequences to both the patient and the physician.[6,7] Older patients, young children, and disabled patients are at the highest risk for wrong-patient surgery, as they may lack the cognitive capacity to understand what they are undergoing.

The overall incidence is difficult to determine because it is often underreported by health care providers, and voluntary incident reporting may greatly underestimate the true incidence by a factor of at least 20.[8,9] Because of this, a few states now have confidential reporting requirements for all wrong-site surgery events or sentinel events. This mandate allows an inquiry (internal and sometimes external) of the circumstances that lead to the event and ways to prevent it.

A review of reports submitted from 2004 to 2006 for wrong-site surgery events and near misses found that more than 40% of these errors reached the patient and nearly 20% resulted in completion of a wrong-side procedure.[6] Most wrong-side surgery involved symmetric anatomic structures, with a 1 in 4 chance that surgeons who work on symmetric structures will be involved in a wrong-site error at some point in their career.[6] Also, anonymous data from the Joint Commission on the Accreditation of Healthcare Organizations (JCAHO) indicated that wrong-site surgery can occur in any setting with 58% occurring in the ambulatory setting, 29% occurring in inpatient operating rooms (ORs), and 13% occurring in emergency departments and intensive care units (ICUs).[10]

Contributing factors to wrong-site surgery include the surgeon specifying the wrong site, not completing a proper time-out, not verifying consent or site markings, inaccurate consents/diagnostic reports/images, or inappropriate patient positioning.[6] The risk of committing these errors is increased in:

Emergent cases when there may not be time to adequately prepare[6]

Cases with unusual physical characteristics, such as in morbidly obese patients or those with physical deformities, which require changes from the norm in patient positioning or equipment[6]

Cases that involve multiple procedures or multiple surgeons, especially if the procedures are on multiple parts of the body[6]

Surgeon characteristics, such as a left-handed surgeon, as most setups are for right-handed surgeons[6]

Communication breakdowns, such as on large surgical teams where team members do not have defined roles or in patients with language barriers.[6,11,12]

In addition, in hospitals with a poor safety culture, mistakes are less likely to be caught before they cause patient harm, as people often do not feel comfortable questioning the primary surgeon.

To reduce the likelihood of these errors, the Joint Commission put together a protocol to standardize the approach to verification of the patient and site. This protocol is organized into 3 phases: the preoperative verification process, marking of the operative site, and a preprocedural briefing time-out before the incision is made (**Fig. 1**).[11–14]

However, despite implementation of these measures, the Pennsylvania Patient Safety Authority saw a trend toward improvement but no significant decrease in the incidence of wrong-side/wrong-site surgery from June 2007 to July 2010. Based on their experiences, they recommended that injection of local or regional anesthetic should be treated as a separate procedure, and that marking of operative sites should always be performed before entering the OR.[15]

Despite the relative rarity of its occurrence, wrong-site/wrong-patient surgery can have catastrophic consequences, and every effort should be made to reduce its incidence. In addition to the safety protocols that are being implemented and improved, the creation of a safety culture and promotion of teamwork is critical to prevent these events from occurring.

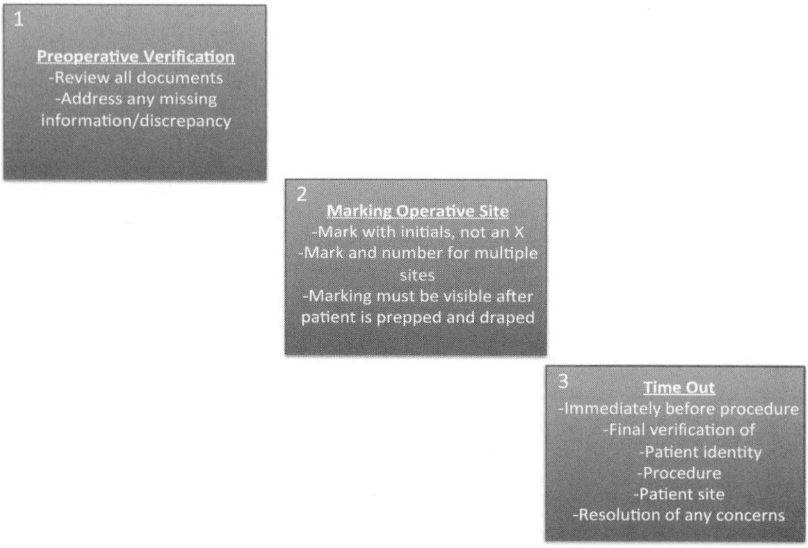

Fig. 1. Protocol for preventing wrong-side/wrong-patient surgery. (*Data from* Refs.[11–14])

PROTOCOLS AND CULTURE CHANGES TO PREVENT ERROR
Barriers to Improved Safety

Among various hospitals, there is up to a sixfold difference in the complication rate,[16] not because the employees working in these hospitals are inherently less skilled or less competent, but because of a poor safety culture. In hospitals with poor safety cultures there are breakdowns in many areas, including a lack of acknowledgment of the high-risk nature of the medical care being performed, a fear of punishment or retaliation if someone reports an error or close call, a lack of communication in large medical teams, and a lack of willingness as an organization to address safety concerns.[8] In one study by the JCAHO, communication was found to be the most important root cause of sentinel events including wrong-site surgeries, contributing to almost 70% of these events.[17] In another study that examined safety cultures in 60 different hospitals, those with poorer safety cultures had increased incidences of wound infection, postoperative sepsis, and postoperative deep vein thrombosis (DVT). It is interesting that postoperative bleeding, which is secondary to a technical error, not a process, did not have an increased incidence across the different hospitals.[16] In light of this, it is clear that creation and perpetuation of a safety culture is a fundamental part of a systems approach to improving patient care.[18]

However, despite attempts at changing culture, some OR environments can be very intimidating for trainees, nurses, and technicians. Such a steep hierarchy combined with a history of disruptive behavior may not promote a culture of speaking up when employees have a safety concern. Studies have suggested that surgeons, in comparison with pilots and other health care professionals, may be less likely to admit that they have made a mistake, that they are at a higher risk for making mistakes than are other specialists, or that stress can have an impact on their decision making.[19,20]

Also, despite a movement in medicine to encourage teamwork and to encourage all members of the surgical team to discuss safety concerns, the steep hierarchy in surgery is still very strong at some medical centers. Although a clear-cut hierarchy is important for patient care in that there must ultimately be one captain of the ship, an atmosphere too intimidating to promote teamwork can result in preventable patient harm. A tense work environment and poor teamwork is often underappreciated by any captain, as demonstrated in a 2006 study on perceptions of teamwork in the OR. This study demonstrated a major disconnect in perceptions among various members of the team. Whereas surgeons rated everyone very highly, nurses rated surgeons very low (**Table 1**). In another study, ICU nurses reported that when compared with doctors, more decisions were made with inadequate input from the nurses, that they were not encouraged to discuss their concerns, and that conflicts were not properly resolved.[21]

Efforts to improve culture are best accomplished through the use of physician-champions who serve as local role models and champions of change.[22] The culture is slowly changing as safety initiatives are being more and more widely implemented, and studies are showing the importance of teamwork and a good safety culture regarding patient care.

Assessment of Safety Culture

To encourage widespread change in safety cultures, it is important to measure a local safety and teamwork culture before and after an intervention to show its impact. The Safety Attitudes Questionnaire (SAQ), which was adapted from the Flight Management Attitudes Questionnaire, is a validated survey instrument used to assess safety culture in different hospitals.[16] The SAQ focuses on 6 different domains including teamwork climate, safety climate, job satisfaction, perceptions of management, stress recognition, and working conditions. In this survey questions focused on the organizational commitment to safety, which has been shown to decrease patients' length of stay and error rates in the ICU.[23]

Within a given hospital, the survey is submitted to all members of the OR team, including surgeons, anesthesiologists, certified registered nurse anesthetists, nurses, and surgical technicians. The safety climate portion of the questionnaire comprises the following:

I am encouraged by my colleagues to report any patient safety concerns I may have
The culture in this clinical area makes it easy to learn from the mistakes of others
Medical errors are handled appropriately in this clinical area
I know the proper channels to direct questions regarding patient safety in this clinical area
I receive appropriate feedback about my performance
I would feel safe being treated here as a patient
In this clinical area, it is difficult to discuss mistakes.

Table 1
Caregivers' ratings of one another's team work

Caregiver position performance rated	Caregiver Position Being Rated			
	Surgeon	Anesthesiologist	Nurse	CRNA
Surgeon	85	84	88	87
Anesthesiologist	70	96	89	92
Nurse	48	63	81	68
CRNA	58	75	76	93

Surgeons rate everyone highly, each caregiver group rates themselves highly, but nurses rate surgeons very low.

From Makary MA, Sexton JP, Freischlag JA, et al. Operating room teamwork among physicians and nurses: teamwork in the eye of the beholder. J Am Coll Surg 2006;202:746; with permission.

Based on this survey, it has been found that safety climate varies dramatically by hospital, but that among various team members in a hospital, perception of safety climate is not significantly different (**Figs. 2** and **3**). Using this survey, hospitals can compare themselves to other hospitals with improved safety climates to determine how to improve. Also, with the push for increasing transparency of outcomes in hospitals, public reporting of SAQ results could further incentivize hospitals to improve their culture, as informed patients would be much less likely to go to the hospital with 16% satisfaction with the safety culture than with 100% satisfaction (see **Fig. 3**).

Improving Teamwork, Communication, and Safety Culture

One of the most effective ways to improve safety culture is to improve communication. In one study there was a 30% rate of communication failure in the OR, with 36% of those failures resulting in an impact on patient safety.[24] In addition to people feeling that they cannot speak up in this environment, the standard workflow in the OR, especially with patient care hand-offs, is particularly prone to loss of important patient information.[25] The introduction of team briefings and debriefings as well as protocols for commonly used procedures has been shown to improve patient safety in the OR and ICU.[26,27]

Preoperative briefings are a discussion of important aspects of the procedure. The briefing can include the names and roles of team members, confirmation of the correct patient/procedure, necessity of antibiotics and if they have been given, the critical steps of the procedure, and potential problems.[27] Such briefings can be tailored to any specialty and are associated with improved safety culture, reduction in incidence of wrong-site/wrong-side surgery, early reporting of equipment problems, fewer OR delays, and reduction in OR costs.[28] Postoperative debriefings are also becoming important by allowing reflection after the case on causes for errors that have occurred and how the procedure could have been run more smoothly. These debriefings can also include a verification of needle and instrument counts and a confirmation of correct labeling of the OR specimen. In addition to reducing the incidence of a retained foreign object, ensuring the correct labeling of the OR specimen can greatly reduce patient harm. In one study 4.3 of 1000 surgical specimens were mislabeled, leading to delays in care, the need for additional biopsy or therapy, and failure to administer appropriate therapy.[29]

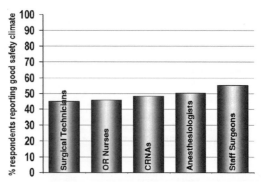

Fig. 2. Safety climate by position. It can be seen that the perception of safety climate is uniform among different surgical team members. CRNA, certified registered nurse anesthetist; OR, operating room. (*From* Makary MA, Sexton JB, Freischlag JA, et al. Patient safety in surgery. Ann Surg 2006;243:628–32; with permission.)

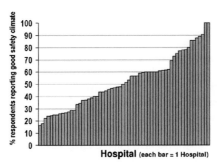

Fig. 3. Safety climate by hospital; each bar represents one hospital. (*From* Makary MA, Sexton JB, Freischlag JA, et al. Patient safety in surgery. Ann Surg 2006;243:628–32; with permission.)

MEASURING QUALITY IN SURGERY
Standardization of Patient Safety Terminology

In addition to bringing patient safety to the forefront of medical innovation, the IOM report standardized the terminology used in patient safety (**Fig. 4**).[1,30] This standardization allowed various agencies to study health care systems using the same language.

Agency for Healthcare Researchers and Quality

The Agency for Healthcare Researchers and Quality (AHRQ) was created in 1989, and is an agency in the Department of Health and Human Services that specializes in research in quality improvement and patient safety, outcomes and effectiveness of care, clinical practice and technology assessment, and health care organization and delivery systems.[8] The research conducted in conjunction with the AHRQ provides evidence-based information on health care outcomes, cost, use, and access, which can be used by health care reformers to make large system-based changes.[8]

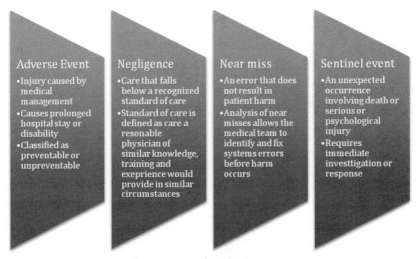

Fig. 4. Characterization of different types of medical errors.

One of the major contributions of the AHRQ was the development of a set of Patient Safety Indicators (PSIs) using hospital inpatient data, initially released in 2003 and revised in 2010. These indicators were developed after a comprehensive literature review, analysis of ICD-9-CM codes, review by a clinician panel, implementation of risk adjustment, and empirical analysis.[31] The 27 indicators provide information from hospital complications and adverse events that can be studied for further systems improvements (**Box 1**). The PSIs are divided into two groups: provider-level indicators and area-level indicators. The provider-level indicators are those whereby a potentially preventable complication occurred in the same hospitalization period during which a patient received initial care. Area-level indicators are specific

---

Box 1
Patient safety indicators (PSIs)

Provider PSIs

- Complications of anesthesia
- Death in low-mortality diagnosis-related groups
- Decubitus ulcer
- Failure to rescue
- Foreign body left during procedure
- Iatrogenic pneumothorax
- Selected infections due to medical care
- Postoperative hip fracture
- Postoperative hemorrhage or hematoma
- Postoperative physiologic and metabolic derangements
- Postoperative respiratory failure
- Postoperative pulmonary embolism or DVT
- Postoperative sepsis
- Postoperative wound dehiscence
- Accidental puncture or laceration
- Transfusion reaction
- Birth trauma: injury to neonate
- Obstetric trauma: vaginal with instrument
- Obstetric trauma: vaginal without instrument
- Obstetric trauma: cesarean delivery

Area-Level PSIs

- Foreign body left during procedure
- Iatrogenic pneumothorax
- Selected infections due to medical care
- Postoperative wound dehiscence
- Accidental puncture or laceration
- Transfusion reaction
- Postoperative hemorrhage or hematoma

PSIs that are also used to assess the total incidence of certain adverse events within geographic areas, during either the initial hospitalization or a related subsequent hospitalization.

These indicators are currently being widely used in hospitals to identify potential safety problems that merit further investigations. As electronic medical records become more standardized, these indicators can be followed to track progress in patient safety at a hospital-specific and nationwide level.

Surgical Care Improvement Project

The Surgical Care Improvement Project (SCIP) is a national partnership of organizations focused on improving surgical care by significantly reducing surgical complications. The organizations involved include the Centers for Medicare and Medicaid Services, the Institute for Healthcare Improvement, JCAHO, the American College of Surgeons, Centers for Disease Control and Prevention, and others.

SCIP has 3 major improvement projects including reduction in infection, prevention of venous thromboembolism (VTE), and cardiac event prevention. Patients who experience these complications have significantly increased length of hospital stay (3–11 day increase), increased hospital cost (up to $18,000 for a thromboembolic event), and increased mortality (median survival decreases by 69%).[32] The evidence-based measures to improve these complications have been shown to reduce infections, VTE, and cardiac events, and are summarized in (**Table 2**).[33]

Surgical-site infections account for up to 15% of all hospital-acquired infections. In addition to significantly improved patient satisfaction, eradication of these infections could save hospitals up to $5000 per patient and reduce extended length of stay by 7 days.[34–36]

Cardiac events are common postoperatively, occurring in up to 5% of patients undergoing noncardiac surgery and up to 34% of those undergoing vascular procedures. Cardiac events can have significant consequences, with myocardial infarctions having a mortality rate of up to 70%. Multiple studies have shown that perioperative β-blockers likely reduce the risk of perioperative ischemia and prevent up to half of fatal cardiac events.[36–38]

Thromboembolic events occur after approximately 25% of all major surgical procedures if prophylaxis is not used, and in orthopedic surgery this number increases to 50%. Studies have shown that using low-dose unfractionated heparin can decrease the risk of fatal pulmonary embolism by up to 50%. Despite multiple studies showing the safety and efficacy of DVT prophylaxis, it continues to be underused or misused.[36,39,40]

Another new SCIP core measure is to publish practitioner performance. With improved transparency in medicine, practitioners can know their own performance and compare it with that of others to improve on individual measures. Also, and more importantly, with improved transparency hospitals can take a systems-based approach to improve patient safety. In addition, patients will be better informed about which hospital to use for their care, thus further incentivizing hospitals to improve.

The SCIP measures are easily implementable, with clear outcome measures to measure their success. With implementation of these measures the potential number of lives saved in the Medicare population alone is greater than 13,000 patients per year.[35] As these are measures are applied to ever widening populations, and as hospital transparency becomes more standard, we will continue to see improvements in the delivery of care to surgical patients.

Although the overall impact of SCIP compliance on improved patient outcomes has been controversial, SCIP will continue to expand and be refined to better capture

Table 2
SCIP measures to reduce rates of infection, venous thromboembolism, and cardiac events

	Performance Measures	Outcome Measures
Infection	Prophylactic antibiotic received within 1 h before surgical incision	Postoperative wound infection diagnosed during initial hospitalization
	Prophylactic antibiotic selection for surgical patients	
	Prophylactic antibiotics discontinued within 24 h after surgery end time	
	Cardiac surgery patients with controlled postoperative 6 AM blood glucose	
	Urinary catheter removed on postoperative day 1 or 2	
	Surgery patients with appropriate hair removal	
	Surgery patients with perioperative temperature management	
Venous thromboembolism (VTE) prophylaxis	Surgery patients with recommended VTE prophylaxis ordered	Intra- or postoperative pulmonary or deep venous embolism diagnosed during initial hospitalization and within 30 d of surgery
	Surgery patients who received appropriate VTE prophylaxis within 24 h before surgery to 24 h after surgery	
Cardiac events	Surgery patients on β-blocker before arrival who received a β-blocker during the perioperative period	Intra- or postoperative acute myocardial infarction diagnosed during initial hospitalization and within 30 d of surgery

meaningful metrics of quality. Never events are more widely accepted as metrics of quality and preventable patient harm. At present, SCIP metrics are transparent but rates of never events are not.

National Surgical Quality Improvement Program

The National Surgical Quality Improvement Program (NSQIP) is a risk-adjusted data-collection mechanism that was created by the Veterans Health Administration (VA) to collect and analyze clinical outcomes data. It allows participating hospitals to collect data and use these data to develop surgical initiatives that improve surgical care.[41] The program is used to compare the performance of participating hospitals, focusing primarily on 30-day morbidity and mortality. Within the first 10 years of its implementation of the program at the VA, the 30-day mortality rate after major surgery decreased by 30% and the 30-day postoperative morbidity decreased by 45%.[16] Testing of the program at 18 non-VA sites from 2001 to 2004 showed feasibility for application of the program in the private sector, and in 2004 it was expanded to more than 200 hospitals to measure outcomes on a large scale.[42]

This program allows hospitals to implement changes and quickly see improvement or lack of improvement against placebo groups at either their own location or other hospitals. As NSQIP use is refined further, we will be able to better understand and fix systems problems and improve patient safety. Some hospitals have expressed eagerness to make their NSQIP outcomes public in the spirit of transparency.

SUMMARY

In the past 15 years, there has been a growing focus on the causes and prevention of medical errors, particularly in surgery. Medical errors are associated with serious patient harm and high health care costs. Although mistakes are inherent in human nature, many errors can be attributed to large and complex health care systems in which care is increasingly fragmented. One of the most important ways to improve health care safety is through improved communication and an improved safety culture. Hospitals with good safety cultures have lower complication rates, and improved patient and staff satisfaction. Transparency in health care is an increasingly recognized means to improve outcomes by allowing the free market to reward hospitals with a strong safety culture, good outcomes, and compliance with evidence-based medicine (ie, checklist compliance). As more data become available regarding strategies that work to improve patient safety and such strategies are more widely implemented, significant improvements in the quality of care that is delivered nationwide should become apparent.

REFERENCES

1. Kohn K, Corrigan J, Donaldson M. To err is human: building a safer health system. Washington, DC: Institute of Medicine, National Academy Press; 1999.
2. Landrigan CP, Parry GJ, Bones CB, et al. Temporal trends in rates of patient harm resulting from medical care. N Engl J Med 2010;363(22):2124–34.
3. Michaels RK, Makary MA, Dahab Y, et al. Achieving the National Quality Forum's "Never Events": prevention of wrong site, wrong procedure, and wrong patient operations. Ann Surg 2007;245(4):526–32.
4. Wrong site surgery. Surgery and anesthesia. Plymouth Meeting (PA): ECRI Institute; 2003;26.
5. Seiden SC, Barach P. Wrong-side/wrong-site, wrong-procedure, and wrong-patient adverse events: are they preventable? Arch Surg 2006;141(9):931–9.
6. Pennsylvania Patient Safety Reporting System (PA-PSRS). Doing the "right" things to correct wrong-site surgery. Patient Safety Advisory 2007;4(1).
7. Kwaan MR, Studdert DM, Zinner MJ, et al. Incidence, patterns, and prevention of wrong-site surgery. Arch Surg 2006;141(4):353–7 [discussion: 357–8].
8. Wald H, Shojania K. Prevention of misidentifications. In: Making Health Care Safer: A Critical Analysis of Patient Safety Practices. Washington, DC: Agency for Healthcare Research and Quality; 2001. p. 491–503.
9. Shojania KG, Duncan BW, McDonald KM, et al. Making health care safer: a critical analysis of patient safety practices. Evid Rep Technol Assess (Summ) 2001;(43): i–x, 1–668.
10. Joint Commission. A follow up review of wrong site surgery. Sentinel event alert 2001;24:1–3.
11. Edwards P. Promoting correct site surgery: a national approach. J Perioper Pract 2006;16(2):80–6.
12. Dunn D. Surgical site verification: a through Z. J Perianesth Nurs 2006;21(5): 317–28 [quiz: 329–31].

13. Joint Commission. Universal protocol for preventing wrong site, wrong procedure, wrong person surgery. Oakbrook Terrace (IL): Joint Commission; 2003.
14. Carney BL. Evolution of wrong site surgery prevention strategies. AORN J 2006; 83(5):1115–8, 1121–22.
15. Pensylvania Patient Safety Reporting System (PA-PSRS). Proceedings Annual Report 2010. Patient safety advisory. Harrisburg (PA) 2010.
16. Makary MA, Sexton JB, Freischlag JA, et al. Patient safety in surgery. Ann Surg 2006;243(5):628–32 [discussion: 632–5].
17. Joint Commission. Sentinel events: evaluating cause and planning improvement. Oakbrook Terrace (IL): Joint Commission of health care organizations; 1998.
18. Vincent C, Moorthy K, Sarker SK, et al. Systems approaches to surgical quality and safety: from concept to measurement. Ann Surg 2004;239(4):475–82.
19. Chan DK, Gallagher TH, Reznick R, et al. How surgeons disclose medical errors to patients: a study using standardized patients. Surgery 2005;138(5): 851–8.
20. Sexton JB, Thomas EJ, Helmreich RL. Error, stress, and teamwork in medicine and aviation: cross sectional surveys. BMJ 2000;320(7237):745–9.
21. Amalberti R, Auroy Y, Berwick D, et al. Five system barriers to achieving ultrasafe health care. Ann Intern Med 2005;142(9):756–64.
22. Makary MA, Sexton JB, Freischlag JA, et al. Operating room teamwork among physicians and nurses: teamwork in the eye of the beholder. J Am Coll Surg 2006;202(5):746–52.
23. Pronovost P, Weast B, Rosenstein B, et al. Implementing and validating a comprehensive unit-based safety program. J Patient Saf 2005;1:33–40.
24. Lingard L, Espin S, Whyte S, et al. Communication failures in the operating room: an observational classification of recurrent types and effects. Qual Saf Health Care 2004;13(5):330–4.
25. Christian CK, Gustafson ML, Roth EM, et al. A prospective study of patient safety in the operating room. Surgery 2006;139(2):159–73.
26. Pronovost PJ, Berenholtz SM, Goeschel CA, et al. Creating high reliability in health care organizations. Health Serv Res 2006;41(4 Pt 2):1599–617.
27. Makary MA, Mukherjee A, Sexton JB, et al. Operating room briefings and wrong-site surgery. J Am Coll Surg 2007;204(2):236–43.
28. Nundy S, Mukherjee A, Sexton JB, et al. Impact of preoperative briefings on operating room delays: a preliminary report. Arch Surg 2008;143(11): 1068–72.
29. Makary MA, Epstein J, Pronovost PJ, et al. Surgical specimen identification errors: a new measure of quality in surgical care. Surgery 2007;141(4):450–5.
30. Woreta TA, Makary MA. Patient safety. In: General Surgery Review. Washington, DC: Ladner-Drysdale; 2008. p. 553.
31. Agency for Healthcare Research, and Quality. Patient safety indicators overview. Rockville (MD): AHRQ; 2006.
32. Bratzler DW. The surgical infection prevention and surgical care improvement projects: promises and pitfalls. Am Surg 2006;72(11):1010–6 [discussion: 1021–30, 1133–48].
33. Available at: http://www.jointcommision.org/surgical_care_improvement_project. Accessed November 21, 2011.
34. Hackney C. Surgical care improvement project. AORN J 2008;87(1):17.
35. Kirkland KB, Briggs JP, Trivette SL, et al. The impact of surgical-site infections in the 1990s: attributable mortality, excess length of hospitalization, and extra costs. Infect Control Hosp Epidemiol 1999;20(11):725–30.

36. Brennan TA, Leape LL, Laird NM, et al. Incidence of adverse events and negligence in hospitalized patients: results of the Harvard Medical Practice Study I. 1991. Qual Saf Health Care 2004;13(2):145–51 [discussion: 151–2].
37. Wallace A, Layug B, Tateo I, et al. Prophylactic atenolol reduces postoperative myocardial ischemia. McSPI Research Group. Anesthesiology 1998;88(1):7–17.
38. Lindenauer PK, Pekow P, Wang K, et al. Perioperative beta-blocker therapy and mortality after major noncardiac surgery. N Engl J Med 2005;353(4):349–61.
39. Collins R, Scrimgeour A, Yusuf S, et al. Reduction in fatal pulmonary embolism and venous thrombosis by perioperative administration of subcutaneous heparin. Overview of results of randomized trials in general, orthopedic, and urologic surgery. N Engl J Med 1988;318(18):1162–73.
40. Bergqvist D, Agnelli G, Cohen AT, et al. Duration of prophylaxis against venous thromboembolism with enoxaparin after surgery for cancer. N Engl J Med 2002;346(13):975–80.
41. Available at: http://www.acsnsqip.org. Accessed November 21, 2011.
42. Khuri SF. Safety, quality, and the National Surgical Quality Improvement Program. Am Surg 2006;72(11):994–8 [discussion: 1021–30, 1133–48].

Hospital-Acquired Infections

Kevin W. Lobdell, MD[a],*, Sotiris Stamou, MD, PhD[b],
Juan A. Sanchez, MD, MPA[c]

KEYWORDS

- Hospital-acquired infection
- Catheter-related bloodstream infection
- Ventilator-associated pneumonia • Surgical site infection
- Catheter-associated urinary tract infection

Health-acquired conditions (HACs) are complications that emanate from a stay in a medical facility. HACs are increasingly scrutinized and apparent because of the staggering gravity of the problem and their threat to sustainability.[1,2] Preventable complications associated with health care in the United States are estimated to cost $88 billion per year.[3] In addition, a 2007 study by Aon suggests that HACs accounted for 12.2% of the health care facilities' total legal liability costs.[4]

The Centers for Medicare & Medicaid Services (CMS) no longer allows additional payment for 4 HACs involving infection. This subset of HACs, health-acquired infection (HAI), is defined by the Centers for Disease Control and Prevention (CDC) as a "localized or systemic condition resulting from an adverse reaction to the presence of infectious agent(s) or its toxin(s)." This article focuses on these HAIs that are well studied, common, and costly (direct, indirect, and intangible). The HAIs reviewed are catheter-related bloodstream infection (CRBSI), ventilator-associated pneumonia (VAP), surgical site infection (SSI), and catheter-associated urinary tract infection (CAUTI). This article excludes discussion of *Clostridium difficile* infections and vancomycin-resistant *Enterococcus*.

The Study on Efficacy of Nosocomial Infection Control elucidated the impact of HAIs when published in 1992. In 2002, the incidence of HAIs was estimated at 1.7 million.[5] More recent data suggest that HAIs may contribute as much as $35 to $45 billion per year.[6] These HAIs are associated with approximately 6% mortality (100,000 deaths per year) in the United States.[6] This total exceeds the mortality attributed to breast and

The authors have nothing to disclose.

[a] Sanger Heart and Vascular Institute, Carolinas HealthCare System, PO Box 32861, Charlotte, NC 28232, USA
[b] Fred and Lena Meijer Heart Center, Michigan State University, 100 Michigan Street North East, Suite 8830, Grand Rapids, MI 49503, USA
[c] Surgery, Saint Mary's Hospital, University of Connecticut, 56 Franklin Street, Waterbury, CT 06706, USA
* Corresponding author.
E-mail address: kevin.lobdell@carolinashealthcare.org

colon cancer combined! The average adjusted length of stay for a hospitalized patient is 5 days, whereas the average length of stay for a patient with an HAI is 22 days.[7]

Fortunately, legislators, CMS, and private health insurance companies are modifying reimbursement schemes to reward quality and disallow additional payments for a growing number of HACs and HAIs. This shift in policy is broadly known as value-based purchasing and integral to the National Quality Strategy (NQS).[8] The NQS aims to improve the overall quality through accessible, safe, reliable, and patient-centered care. In addition, the NQS intends to address the affordability of health care and result in improved health of individuals and communities.

Transparency, through public reporting, compliments the aforementioned alteration in incentives. Various public reporting sites and entities exist, including Hospital Compare, HealthGrades, US News & World Report, Thomson Reuters, and various federal, state, and privately sponsored efforts. The prototype for leadership in transparency is the Society of Thoracic Surgeons partnership with Consumers Union to voluntarily report process and outcome measures associated with adult cardiac surgery.[9] This leadership is commendable and provides a template for other societies to define and report on the quality of their efforts.

To ascertain quality, health care teams must do the right things by using evidence-based medicine (EBM) guidelines. Information technology (IT), through computer order entry and decision support, supports EBM. Simultaneously, health care teams must ascertain that they are doing things right by continuously improving performance and reliability. Goal sheets, bundles, checklists, and multidisciplinary care are integral to high performance in today's dynamic, competitive, and transparent environment.[10–16]

Education, including novel simulation methods, is a mainstay in performance improvement. A thorough knowledge of microbiological factors associated with HAIs (methicillin-resistant *Staphylococcus aureus* [MRSA] and methicillin-resistant *Staphylococcus epidermidis* [MRSE] and multidrug-resistant [MDR] gram-negative aerobes) is necessary. The adoption of affordable innovative technology and processes are also central to the quality improvement journey. IT can catalyze the process of data management and surveillance by assisting in the collection of accurate real-time data. These data should be rapidly analyzed and reviewed by "learning" health care teams who strive to provide their patients with high-quality care.

CRBSI
Definition and Diagnosis

CRBSI is a clinical definition used when tests implicate the catheter as the source of the infection. CRBSI is commonly suspected when a patient with an intravascular catheter has local and/or systemic signs/symptoms consistent with infection and no other source of infection. For example, a central venous catheter (CVC) may have erythema, induration, purulence, or tenderness at the insertion site. Alternatively, a patient with a CVC may have only fever and/or leukocytosis. A central line–associated bloodstream infection (CLABSI) may be defined as a bloodstream infection (BSI) in a patient who had a CVC within the 48-hour period before the development of the BSI and is not related to a remote infection.[17]

The offending organism is preferentially cultured from the catheter tip, although it may be cultured from the site, from blood through the catheter, or through peripheral blood culture. Methods used to culture from catheter tip include sonication or roll plating. Other methods to assist in diagnosis include differential time of blood culture positivity, acridine orange leukocyte cytospin, and paired quantitative blood culture.[18–20]

Epidemiology and Economics

Catheter use is prevalent in modern health care, particularly in the intensive care unit (ICU) setting. CVC use in the United States may exceed 15 million catheter-days each year.[21] CRBSIs have been estimated at 250,000 cases per year.[22] CLABSIs predominate the CRBSIs, and estimates range from 80,000 to 92,000 cases per year.[6,23] When CRBSIs are expressed in rate per 1000 catheter-days, the range may vary from 1.6 to 6.8.[24,25]

Peripheral venous catheters seem to incur fewer clinically apparent infections (0.6 per 1000 catheter-days) than nontunneled CVCs (2.3 per 1000 catheter-days). Rates of infection, expressed in rate per 1000 catheter-days, are as follows: peripherally inserted CVCs, 0.4; subcutaneous central venous ports, 0.2; cuffed/tunneled CVCs, 1.2; arterial catheter, 2.9; pulmonary artery catheter, 5.5; cuffed hemodialysis, 1.1; and noncuffed hemodialysis, 2.8.[25]

Average attributable costs of CLABSI estimates range from $25,849 to $45,000 per case.[6,26] These CLABSIs are estimated to contribute $670,000,000 to $4,000,000,000 in hospital costs each year in the United States.[6,26] Mortality attributable to CRBSI ranges from 0% to 17%.[27–29]

Risk Factors and Mechanisms

Risk factors for CRBSI include, but are not limited to, type of catheter (tunneled, nontunneled, venous, arterial), type of port,[30] location, securing methods, duration of use, host factors (age, severity of illness, immune deficiency), transfusions of blood products and total parenteral nutrition, techniques to place and maintain catheters, and location of care.[31,32]

CRBSI is most commonly extraluminal. The extraluminal infections originate from microbes colonizing skin at the site of catheter insertion or hematogenous seeding. CRBSIs may also originate intraluminally from accessing catheters and infusates.

Microbiology

Organisms most commonly associated with CRBSI include *Staphylococcus epidermidis*, *Staphylococcus aureus*, *Enterococci*, various gram-negative bacilli, and *Candida albicans*. Antimicrobial resistance is a growing concern in many of the causative organisms. Most CRBSIs are monomicrobial, but polymicrobial infections are not uncommon.

Treatment

Catheter removal is fundamental to treatment of CRBSI. Exception to this rule relates to the type of organism (*Staphylococcus epidermidis*), rapid clearance of bacteremia, importance of device, and lack of suitable alternatives. For example, a hemodialysis catheter infected with *Staphylococcus epidermidis* may be appropriately and adequately treated with antibiotics. *Staphylococcus aureus*, gram-negative bacteria, and fungi should not be treated with catheter retention and intravenous antibiotics (or lock therapy). Similarly, rewiring infected catheters should be the exception rather than the rule in treating CRBSIs.

Although antibiotic therapy is routine and appropriate, the duration of therapy is variable. Commonly, uncomplicated CVC infections have antibiotic therapy targeted at the offending organism for 7 to 10 days. Complicated infections (including infected thrombus, endocarditis, osteomyelitis) may require 4 to 8 weeks of antibiotic treatment.

Prevention and Quality Improvement

Improving the rate of CRBSI, with the goal of eradicating them, is increasingly a priority for health care teams and institutions. Fundamentals of improving include education and training,[33,34] appropriate staffing,[35] and use of process checklists and procedure carts.[36]

The operator's choice of site, hand hygiene, aseptic technique and use of 2% chlorhexidine skin preparation, and maximal sterile barrier are priorities in preventing CRBSI.[23] Meticulous and appropriate catheter site care is vital. Chlorhexidine-impregnated sponges and antimicrobial catheters have been associated with reduced rates of CRBSI and should be considered in any comprehensive attack on improving HAIs.[25,37] Antimicrobial ointments, flushes, and locks may also play select roles in strategies designed to mitigate the risk of CRBSI.[25,38] Routine replacement of CVC is not recommended as a strategy to mitigate risk of CRBSI.[23] Standard operating procedure should be developed for replacement of administration sets (typically every 4 to 7 days).[23] Tubing should be changed within 24 hours of initiation of blood product and/or total parenteral nutrition.[23]

Comprehensive strategies to improve the rate of CRBSIs have appropriately garnered considerable attention and resources.[39] More recent evaluation of the concerted pioneering Keystone Intensive Care Unit Project suggests that the effort is sustainable and replicable.[40,41]

Real-time data collection, analysis, and monitoring and management of operations are also vital to performance improvement.[42]

VAP
Definition and Diagnosis

VAP is a pneumonia that is associated with mechanical ventilation. Definitions vary amongst databases, registries, and clinical investigations. The literature must be interpreted carefully with an appreciation of the nuances of each study's definitions and design.

Symptoms and signs vary but commonly include malaise, fever, chills, purulent respiratory secretions, rhonchi, leukocytosis, infiltrate on plain chest radiograph, and impaired oxygenation and ventilation. Blood culture results may be positive because of VAP and should accompany the diagnostic evaluation. Commonly used diagnostic modalities include Gram stain, nonquantitative or quantitative tracheal aspirate cultures, protected suction cultures, and bronchoscopic cultures. Bronchoalveolar lavage has been extensively studied and has many proponents.

Often a patient suffering from VAP exhibits the systemic inflammatory response syndrome (SIRS). Patients with SIRS may benefit from intensive monitoring and judicious administration of fluids as well as inotrope and/or vasopressor support. A comprehensive view including evaluation of remote organ function (liver, kidney, heart, and so forth) should be routine.

Epidemiology and Economics

VAP is estimated to afflict approximately 52,000 patients per year in the United States.[6] Recently, VAP was determined to complicate the course of 8% to 28% of mechanically ventilated patients,[43] although some ICUs are now reporting eradication of VAP.

VAP is associated with increased ICU and hospital lengths of stay as well as prolonged mechanical ventilation. Average attributable cost estimates of VAP range from $12,000 to more than $40,000 per case.[6,43,44] Mortality attributable to VAP ranges from 24% to 76%.[45] VAP is the HAI associated with the highest risk of mortality.

Risk Factors and Mechanisms

Risk for VAP is well studied, and many variables have been suggested to increase the risk of VAP. Host factors associated with an increased risk of VAP include age, male gender, neurologic impairment, and muscular weakness.[46] Other variables include duration of ventilation, reintubation, aspiration, severity of illness, adult respiratory distress syndrome, cardiac disease, paralytic agents, tracheostomy, surgery, trauma, and burns.[44,46,47]

Microbiology

Aerobic gram-negative bacilli account for approximately 60% of VAPs.[43] These aerobic gram-negative bacilli are commonly *Pseudomonas aeruginosa*, *Acinetobacter* species, *Proteus* species, *Escherichia coli*, *Klebsiella* species, and *Haemophilus influenza*. Staphylococcus aureus seems to represent 20% to 30% of VAPs and is increasing in incidence. Fungi, most commonly *Candida* species, are often cultured in patients thought to have VAP, but lung biopsy with yeast or pseudohyphae is diagnostic. Viruses, such as cytomegalovirus, are typically associated with VAP in immunosuppressed patients (transplantation, neoplasia, immune deficiency syndromes, and so forth).

Antibiotic resistance is a growing problem in gram-negative aerobes as well as in *Staphylococcus* species.

Treatment

A high index of suspicion must be maintained to rapidly diagnose VAP. Although reliable techniques for diagnosis exist, early empiric therapy should be directed at common pathogens seen in the local environment while considering idiosyncratic host factors (history, known diseases, immunosuppression, and so forth). Antimicrobial therapy should be tailored to the cultures and clinical situation as a part of de-escalation strategies.

Complications of VAP can include lung abscess and thoracic empyema. Lung abscess may require tube drainage, whereas parapneumonic effusions and thoracic empyema may require surgical intervention (thoracostomy tube drainage, thoracoscopy/thoracotomy, decortication, and so forth).

Prevention and Quality Improvement

Eliminating VAP is a common goal for teams caring for patients supported with mechanical ventilation. Cornerstones for performance improvement include education about VAP and risk mitigation, training (to include set up, maintenance, and cleaning of respiratory equipment), hand cleansing, VAP bundle,[48] and surveillance.

The VAP bundles include strategies to reduce the risk of aspirating secretions with a high bacterial load (elevating the head of bed 30°–45°, avoiding gastric distention, antiseptic oropharyngeal care, use of cuffed endotracheal tubes and in-line suctioning, and judicious use of gastric acid suppression) paired with daily sedation vacations and spontaneous breathing trials. Endotracheal tubes designed to assist subglottic suctioning may be useful.

Surveillance should include monitoring and management to ascertain compliance with vital processes as well as evaluation of outcomes and transparency.

Selective use of noninvasive positive pressure ventilation, which is efficacious and increasingly used, avoids the use of positive pressure mechanical ventilation and may be advantageous in reducing the risk of VAP.[49]

SSI
Definition and Diagnosis

There are 4 common definitions of SSI[50]:

(1) The 1992 CDC definition that includes observation of 16 wound or patient characteristics and has 2 additional criteria (surgeon's diagnosis of infection and culture of microorganisms from the wound).[51] In addition, the classification includes depths of infection, including superficial, deep, and organ space
(2) Nosocomial Infection National Surveillance Scheme modification of the CDC definition that requires positive culture result of tissue or fluid but excludes swabs
(3) Purulent wound drainage
(4) ASEPSIS scoring method that provides a numerical score related to the severity of wound infection using objective criteria based on wound appearance and the clinical consequences of the infection[52]

Various databases, registries, and collaboratives may also have definitions specific for specialty or surgical type.

Epidemiology and Economics

SSIs are prevalent, accounting for approximately 15% of HAIs. Surgical procedures have been estimated at more than 45,000,000 per year in the United States[53] and are associated with 290,485 to 400,000 SSIs per year.[6,54] SSIs occur in 2% to 5% of patients after clean extra-abdominal operations and in up to 20% of patients undergoing intra-abdominal operations.[55] Risk of SSI increases from clean to clean-contaminated through contaminated and dirty classifications as well as varies between specialties (cardiac surgery, orthopedics, general surgery, and so forth). SSIs contribute significantly to morbidity and mortality, and the economic impact of SSI is tremendous. The costs attributable to SSI are $11,087 to $29,443 per case and as much as $3,450,000,000 to 10,000,000,000 per year in the United States.[6]

Surveillance[54,56] is fundamental to any description of SSIs. Consistent interpretation must accompany common definition as well as precision to differentiate attack rates. Quantitative antibiotic exposure, using pharmacy data, is a useful surveillance method. Questionnaires have been used but are cumbersome and inaccurate. Administrative data may contribute invaluably to postdischarge surveillance. Similarly, health information exchanges may bolster surveillance.

Risk Factors and Mechanisms

Most SSIs result from microbes invading the surgical wound at the time of operation.

Host factors associated with SSI include age, diabetes mellitus, nutritional status, body mass index, immunosuppression, MRSA carriers, chronic obstructive pulmonary disease, and hepatic or renal failure.[57–60] Status of operation (elective, urgent, emergent, and salvage) can also affect the rate of SSI. Additional factors of SSI include (but are not limited to) length of preoperative stay in a health care facility, technique of hair removal, antimicrobial skin cleansing methods, draping, sterile technique (hand washing, air flow in operating rooms, maintenance of sterility), surgical technique (electrocautery, suture types, hemostatic agents, bone wax), duration and type of operation, and antibiotic choice, timing, and duration.[57,58,61–64] Perioperative euglycemia is thought to be important in reducing the risk of deep sternal wound infections associated with adult cardiac surgery,[65] although the role of euglycemia is less clear with other procedures.

Microbiology

Most SSIs in clean surgical procedures involve *Staphylococcus* species from the exogenous environment or the patient's skin flora, although a significant percentage of clean cases develop SSI because of gram-negative organisms.

Pathogens in clean-contaminated (gastrointestinal, gynecologic, and respiratory tracts have been entered), contaminated, and dirty SSIs mirror the endogenous microflora of the surgical site and/or resected organ.

Despite a growing problem of antimicrobial resistance (eg, MRSA, MRSE, and MDR gram-negative aerobes), the incidence and distribution of the pathogens isolated from SSIs have been relatively constant.

Treatment

Opening infected wounds, supplemented with local wound care, is a traditional and well-tested therapy for SSI. Targeted parenteral antibiotics supplement local wound care as indicated (cutaneous erythema; involvement of surrounding soft tissues, bone, and devices). Wound sponges with suction (vacuum-assisted closure [VAC]) have gained popularity. VACs assist in wound care maintenance as well as in accelerating treatment and closure of many infected wounds. Various muscle flaps can assist in bringing additional blood flow to infected surgical sites and obliterating space, which can prevent adequate treatment (eg, deep sternal wound infections and postpneumonectomy empyema).

Prevention and Quality Improvement

Many efforts have been reported to reduce the rate of death and complications associated with surgery and specifically SSI. The noteworthy and efficacious efforts include the Veterans Affairs Administration National Surgical Quality Improvement Project[66]; Surgical Infection Prevention project, which was created by CMS in collaboration with the CDC[67]; and the Surgical Care Improvement Project, which began in 2003 through the CMS and the CDC (with 10 organizations on the steering committee and many others collaborating).

Fundamentals of performance improvement in SSI include education, training, management of vital processes, surveillance, and transparency. Any effort directed at improving the rate of SSI should focus attention on hand cleansing, MRSA screening, modification of host risk factors, timing of operation, hair removal and skin preparation, operating room sterility, antimicrobials (nasal application of mupirocin, choice, timing, and duration of antibiotics, bowel preparation regimens, and so forth), operative technique and surgical sites, and normothermia when applicable.

CAUTI
Definition and Diagnosis

Generally, more than 100,000 colony-forming units (CFU)/ml of urine is thought to be diagnostic of a urinary tract infection, although smaller numbers of organisms can rapidly become problematic if not treated or suppressed in a hospitalized patient treated with an indwelling urinary catheter. As a result, CAUTI is commonly defined as more than 1000 to 10,000 CFU/mL of urine. CAUTI is the second most common cause of bacteremia in hospitalized patients.[68]

Epidemiology and Economics

One in 5 hospitalized patients has a urinary catheter placed,[69] and urinary catheter use is almost ubiquitous in ICUs.[70,71] CAUTI is the most common HAI and is estimated to occur in 449,334 cases per year in the United States.[6] The risk of bacteriuria increases by 5% each day a patient has an indwelling urinary catheter,[72] although most CAUTIs are asymptomatic and not associated with urosepsis. Systemic therapy for asymptomatic bacteriuria should be reserved for high-risk (immunosuppressed) patients. Screening for bacteriuria can be associated with increased use of antimicrobials and the development of drug resistance.

Average attributable costs of CAUTI estimates range from $749 to $832 per case.[6] CAUTIs in the United States are estimated to contribute $390,000,000 to $450,000,000 annually in hospital costs. Mortality attributable to CAUTI differs amongst investigations and their risk modeling but currently is thought to approach zero.[73]

CAUTI is an enormous reservoir for antimicrobial-resistant MDR gram-negative aerobes. Cross infection with MDR gram-negative aerobes has been documented.

Risk Factors and Mechanisms

Most commonly, microbes contaminate the urinary tract extraluminally (external contamination and capillary action).[74] Intraluminal sources are also important (through breaks in the system or reflux of collected urine). Biofilm,[75] a host protein and microbial exoglycocalyx matrix, may be responsible for both intraluminal and extraluminal contamination. Organisms responsible for CAUTI are commonly associated with perineal and colonic flora. In addition, CAUTI may originate from the hands of health care workers during placement or maintenance practices.

Host factor risks for CAUTI include female gender, diabetes mellitus, renal insufficiency, malnutrition, and remote sites of infection. Additional risk factors include prolonged catheterization, manipulation of the urinary tract and ureteral stents, and reflux of urine from collecting bag. Long-term antimicrobial therapy is a risk for development of drug-resistant CAUTI.

Microbiology

Escherichia coli, Enterococci, Pseudomonas aeruginosa, Klebsiella and Enterobacter species, and Candida species are most common. Low levels of bacteriuria and funguria can multiply and result in CAUTI within 24 to 48 hours.[76]

Treatment

Catheter removal (or change if ongoing use is necessary) and appropriate targeted antimicrobial therapy is the standard treatment. Antimicrobial solution irrigation has been documented to increase the rate of CAUTI and is avoided with the exception of select fungal CAUTIs.

Prevention and Quality Improvement

Education should focus on CAUTI awareness, appropriate use of urinary catheters (avoidance and alternatives), risks, and removal protocols. Training should be directed at sterile insertion technique, maintenance practices including dependent drainage to prevent reflux, and preventing breaks in the collection system. Insertion should always include sterile gloves, fenestrated drape, and thorough skin preparation with chlorhexidine or povidone-iodine solution. The evaluation of a bladder bundle is currently underway.[77] Surveillance is a mainstay in CAUTI prevention efforts.

About 25% to 75% of CAUTIs are estimated to be avoidable.[69] Protocols for removal are generally simple and successful. A recent study of 600 hospitals demonstrated that fewer than 10% of hospitals use catheter removal reminders or stop-orders. In addition, many institutions (56%) do not have a monitoring system for urinary catheters and nearly 75% do not monitor duration of use.[78] One multidisciplinary effort in 3

ICUs, with guidelines for appropriate catheter placement and a nurse-driven protocol to remove unnecessary catheters without a physician order, reported CAUTI rates decreased by 17% to 45%, with postintervention CAUTI rates of 8.3 to 11.2 per 1000 catheter-days.[79]

Bladder scanning can reduce the rate of urinary catheter placement and hence the rate of CAUTI.

Novel technology includes medicated catheters (through antimicrobial coating and impregnation). The efficacy varies depending on organism, and the value is also variable.

Vaccines against common and MDR nosocomial organisms associated with CAUTI (and other HAIs) hold promise but are not clinically relevant at present.

SUMMARY

HAIs are prevalent and a tremendous burden to patients, the health care system, and the nation's scarce resources. There is an extensive body of literature related to the modifiable risks associated with HAIs.

The ability to incorporate and replicate evidence-based practices into various institutions with their unique cultures is well studied but remains challenging.[80] Understanding human factors, such as the principles of change, organizational behavior and crew resource management, quality, and safety, is vital to successful performance improvement and combating risk.

Novel technologies will accelerate the diagnosis, treatment, and prevention of HAIs. Various IT solutions have accelerated institutional learning by providing health care teams with accurate real-time data and analysis.

Standardizing definitions, sharing information amongst various databases and registries, and health information exchanges are priorities for the US health care system and in combating HAIs.

REFERENCES

1. Healthcare-associated infections—the burden. Available at: http://www.cdc.gov/HAI/burden.html. Accessed July 19, 2011.
2. Centers for Medicare and Medicaid Services. New information to improve patient safety at America's hospitals. Available at: http://www.gha.org/pha/provider/publications/newsletter/041111/resources/HACsFinal.pdf. Accessed July 19, 2011.
3. Fuller R, McCullough E, Bao M, et al. Estimating the costs of potentially preventable hospital acquired complications. Health Care Financ Rev 2009;30(4):17–32. Available at: http://www.cms.gov/HealthCareFinancingReview/downloads/09SummerPg17. pdf. Accessed July 19, 2011.
4. Zieger A. Never events major factor in hospital liability costs. Available at: http://www.fiercehealthcare.com/story/study-never-events-major-factor-hospital-liability-costs/2008-10-01?cmp-id=EMC-NL-FH&dest=FH. Accessed July 19, 2011.
5. Klevens M, Edwards J, Richards C, et al. Estimating health care-associated infections and deaths in U.S. hospitals. Public Health Rep 2007;122:160–7.
6. Scott D. The direct medical costs of HAIs in US hospitals and the benefits of prevention. Available at: http://www.cdc.gov/ncidod/dhqp/pdf/Scott_CostPaper. pdf. Accessed July 19, 2011.
7. Savage B, Segal M, Alexander D. The cost of healthcare associated infections. Available at: https://www2.gehealthcare.com/doccart/public?guid=56c1c4429f811310VgnVCM10000024dd1403. Accessed July 19, 2011.

8. National Strategy for Quality Improvement in Health Care. U.S. Department of Health and Human Services (HHS). Available at: http://www.healthcare.gov/center/reports/quality03212011a.html. Accessed July 19, 2011.

9. Available at: www.consumerreports.org/health/resources/pdf/society-of-thoracic-surgeons/Heart-Surgery-Ratings-Background-and-Methodology.pdf. Accessed November 18, 2011.

10. Stamou S, Camp S, Stiegel R, et al. Quality improvement program decreases mortality after cardiac surgery. J Thorac Cardiovasc Surg 2008;136(2):494–9.

11. Stamou S, Camp S, Reams M, et al. Continuous quality improvement program and major morbidity after cardiac surgery. Am J Cardiol 2008;102(6):772–7.

12. Camp S, Stamou S, Stiegel R, et al. Quality improvement program increases early tracheal extubation rate and decreases pulmonary complications and resource utilization after cardiac surgery. J Card Surg 2009;24:414–23.

13. Lobdell K, Stiegel R, Reames M, et al. Quality improvement and cardiac critical care. Ann Thorac Surg 2010;89:1701.

14. Lobdell K, Stamou S, Mishra A, et al. Multidisciplinary rounds: the work, not more work. Ann Thorac Surg 2010;89:1010.

15. Lobdell K. Value creation in cardiac surgery using the Toyota Production System. Ann Thorac Surg 2011;92:775–6.

16. Gawande A. The checklist. The New Yorker. Available at: http://www.newyorker.com/reporting/2007/12/10/071210fa_fact_gawande. Accessed July 19, 2011.

17. Horan T, Andrus M, Dudeck MA. Surveillance definition of health care-associated infection and criteria for specific types of infections in the acute care setting. Am J Infect Control 2008;36:309–32.

18. Raad I, Hanna H, Alakech B, et al. Differential time to positivity: a useful method for diagnosing catheter-related bloodstream infections. Ann Intern Med 2004; 140(1):18–26.

19. Bong J, Kite P, Ammori B, et al. The use of a rapid in situ test in the detection of central venous catheter-related bloodstream infection: a prospective study. JPEN J Parenter Enteral Nutr 2003;27(2):146–50.

20. Safdar N, Fine J, Maki D. Meta-analysis: methods for diagnosing intravascular device–related bloodstream infection. Ann Intern Med 2005;142(6):451–66.

21. Mermel L. Prevention of intravascular catheter-related infections. Ann Intern Med 2000;132:391–402.

22. Maki D, Kluger D, Crnich C. The risk of bloodstream infection in adults with different intravascular devices: a systematic review of 200 published prospective studies. Mayo Clin Proc 2006;81:1159–71.

23. O'Grady N, Alexander M, Burns L, et al. Guidelines for the prevention of intravascular catheter-related infections, 2011. Available at: http://www.cdc.gov/hicpac/pdf/guidelines/bsi-guidelines-2011.pdf. Accessed July 19, 2011.

24. Edwards J, Peterson K, Andrus M, et al. National Healthcare Safety Network (NHSN) Report, data summary for 2006. Am J Infect Control 2007;35:290–301.

25. Crnich C, Maki D. The promise of novel technology for the prevention of intravascular device–related bloodstream infection. I. Pathogenesis and short-term devices. Clin Infect Dis 2002;34:1232–42.

26. O'Grady N, Alexander M, Dellinger E, et al. Guidelines for the prevention of intravascular catheter-related infections. MMWR Recomm Rep 2002;51:1–29. Available at: www.cdc.gov/mmwr/preview/mmwrhtml/rr5110al.htm. Accessed July 19, 2011.

27. Digiovine B, Chenoweth C, Watts C, et al. The attributable mortality and costs of primary nosocomial bloodstream infections in the intensive care unit. Am J Respir Crit Care Med 1999;160(3):976–81.

28. Diekema D, Beekmann S, Chapin K, et al. Epidemiology and outcome of nosocomial and community-onset bloodstream infection. J Clin Microbiol 2003;41: 3655–60.
29. Blot S, Depuydt P, Annemans L. Clinical and economic outcomes in critically ill patients with nosocomial catheter-related bloodstream infections. Clin Infect Dis 2005;41:1591–8.
30. Maragakis L, Bradley K, Song X, et al. Increased catheter-related bloodstream infection rates after the introduction of a new mechanical valve intravenous access port. Infect Control Hosp Epidemiol 2006;27:1.
31. Charalambous C, Swoboda S, Dick J, et al. Risk factors and clinical impact of central line infections in the surgical intensive care unit. Arch Surg 1998;133:1241.
32. Hanna H, Raad I. Blood products: a significant risk factor for long-term catheter-related bloodstream infections in cancer patients. Infect Control Hosp Epidemiol 2001;22(2):165–6.
33. Warren D, Zack J, Mayfield J, et al. The effect of an education program on the incidence of central venous catheter-associated bloodstream infection in a medical ICU. Chest 2004;126:1612–8.
34. Coopersmith C, Rebmann T, Zack J, et al. Effect of an education program on decreasing catheter-related bloodstream infections in the surgical intensive care unit. Crit Care Med 2002;30(1):59–64.
35. Robert J, Fridkin S, Blumberg H, et al. The influence of the composition of the nursing staff on primary bloodstream infection rates in a surgical intensive care. Infect Control Hosp Epidemiol 2000;21(1):12–7.
36. Berenholtz S, Pronovost P, Lipsett P, et al. Eliminating catheter-related bloodstream infections in the intensive care unit. Crit Care Med 2004;32(10):2014–20.
37. Darouiche R, Raad I, Heard S, et al. A comparison of two antimicrobial-impregnated central venous catheters. N Engl J Med 1999;340:1–8.
38. Wilcox T. Catheter-related bloodstream infections. Semin Intervent Radiol 2009; 26(2):139–43. DOI: 10.1055/s-0029-1222458.
39. Pronovost P, Needham D, Berenholtz S, et al. An intervention to decrease catheter-related bloodstream infections in the ICU. N Engl J Med 2006;355:2725–32.
40. Pronovost P. Interventions to decrease catheter-related bloodstream infections in the ICU: the Keystone Intensive Care Unit Project. Am J Infect Control 2008; 36(10). S171.e1–S171.e5.
41. Pronovost P, Goeschel C, Colantuoni E, et al. Sustaining reductions in catheter related bloodstream infections in Michigan intensive care units: observational study. BMJ 2010;340:c309.
42. Wall R, Ely E, Elasy T, et al. Using real time process measurements to reduce catheter related bloodstream infections in the intensive care unit. Qual Saf Health Care 2005;14:295–302.
43. Shorr A, Kollef M. Ventilator-associated pneumonia: insights from recent clinical trials. Chest 2005;128:583–91.
44. Rello J, Ollendorf D, Oster G, et al. Epidemiology and outcomes of ventilator-associated pneumonia in a large US database. Chest 2002;122:2115–21.
45. Chastre J, Fagon J. Ventilator-associated pneumonia. Am J Respir Crit Care Med 2002;165:867–903.
46. Cook D, Kollef H. Risk factors for ICU-acquired pneumonia. JAMA 1998;279: 1605–6.
47. Cook D, Walter S, Cook R, et al. Incidence of and risk factors for ventilator-associated pneumonia in critically ill patients. Ann Intern Med 1998;129(6): 433–40.

48. Coffin S, Klompas M, Classen D, et al. Strategies to prevent ventilator-associated pneumonia in acute care hospitals. Infect Control Hosp Epidemiol 2008;29:94.
49. Girou E, Brun-Buisson C, Taille S, et al. Secular trends in nosocomial infections and mortality associated with noninvasive ventilation in patients with exacerbation of COPD and pulmonary edema. JAMA 2003;290(22):2985–91.
50. Wilson A, Gibbons C, Reeves B, et al. Surgical wound infection as a performance indicator: agreement of common definitions of wound. BMJ 2004;329:720, 10.1136 1–5.
51. Horan T, Gaynes R, Martone W, et al. CDC definitions of nosocomial surgical site infections. Infect Control Hosp Epidemiol 1992;13(10):606–8.
52. Russell B, Krukowski M. The measurement and monitoring of surgical adverse events. Health Technol Assess 2001;5(22):1–194.
53. Owings M, Kozak L. Ambulatory and inpatient procedures in the United States. Vital Health Stat 13 1998;(139):1–119.
54. Platt R, Yokoe D, Sands K. Automated methods for surveillance of surgical site infections. Emerg Infect Dis 2001;7(2):212–6.
55. Bratzler D, Houck P, Richards C, et al. Use of antimicrobial prophylaxis for major surgery: baseline results from the National Surgical Infection Prevention Project. Arch Surg 2005;140:174–82.
56. Sands K, Yokoe D, Hooper D, et al. Detection of postoperative surgical-site infections: comparison of health plan–based surveillance with hospital-based programs. Infect Control Hosp Epidemiol 2003;24(10):740–3.
57. Gottrup F, Melling A, Hollander D. An overview of surgical site infections: aetiology, incidence and risk factors. EWMA J 2005. Available at: worldwidewounds.com.
58. Neumayer L, Hosokawa P, Itani K, et al. Multivariable predictors of postoperative surgical site infection after general and vascular surgery: results from the patient safety in surgery study. J Am Coll Surg 2007;204(6):1178–87.
59. Manian F, Meyer P, Setzer J, et al. Surgical site infections associated with methicillin-resistant Staphylococcus aureus: do postoperative factors play a role? Clin Infect Dis 2003;36:863–8.
60. Muñoz P, Hortal J, Giannella M, et al. Nasal carriage of S. aureus increases the risk of surgical site infection after major heart surgery. J Hosp Infect 2008; 68(1):25–31.
61. Ridgeway S, Wilson J, Charlet A, et al. Infection of the surgical site after arthroplasty of the hip. J Bone Joint Surg Br 2005;87(6):844–50.
62. Russo P, Epi G, Spelman D. A new surgical-site infection risk index using risk factors identified by multivariate analysis for patients undergoing coronary artery bypass graft surgery. Infect Control Hosp Epidemiol 2002;23(7):372–6.
63. Leong G, Wilson J, Charlett A. Duration of operation as a risk factor for surgical site infection: comparison of English and US data. J Hosp Infect 2006;63: 255–62.
64. Hawn M, Itani K, Gray S, et al. Association of timely administration of prophylactic antibiotics for major surgical procedures and surgical site infection. J Am Coll Surg 2008;206(5):814–9.
65. Furnary A, Zerr K, Grunkemeier G, et al. Continuous intravenous insulin infusion reduces the incidence of deep sternal wound infection in diabetic patients after cardiac surgical procedures. Ann Thorac Surg 1999;67(2):352–60.
66. Khuri S, Daley J, Henderson W, et al. The Department of Veterans Affairs NSQIP: the first national validated, outcome-based, risk-adjusted and peer-controlled program for the measurement and enhancement of the quality of surgical care. Ann Surg 1998;228:491–507.

67. Surgical infection prevention. Available at: www.medqic.org/sip. Accessed November 18, 2011.
68. Maki DG. Nosocomial bacteremia. An epidemiologic overview. Am J Med 1981; 70:719–32.
69. Saint S, Meddings J, Calfee D, et al. Catheter-associated urinary tract infection and the Medicare rule changes. Ann Intern Med 2009;150(12):877–84.
70. Richards M, Edwards J, Culver D, et al. Nosocomial infections in combined medical-surgical intensive care units in the United States. Infect Control Hosp Epidemiol 2000;21(8):510–5.
71. Vincent J, Bihari D, Suter P, et al. The prevalence of nosocomial infection in intensive care units in Europe: results of the European prevalence of infection in intensive care study. JAMA 1995;274:639–44.
72. Maki D, Tambyah P. Engineering out the risk for infection with urinary catheters. Emerg Infect Dis 2001;7(2):342–7.
73. Clech C, Schwebel C, Francais A, et al. Does catheter-associated urinary tract infection increase mortality in critically ill patients? Infect Control Hosp Epidemiol 2007;28:12.
74. Tambyah P, Halvorson K, Maki D. A prospective study of pathogenesis of catheter-associated urinary tract infections. Mayo Clin Proc 1999;74:131–6.
75. Trautner B, Darouiche R. Role of biofilm in catheter-associated urinary tract infection. Am J Infect Control 2004;32(3):177–83.
76. Stark R, Maki D. Bacteriuria in the catheterized patient. N Engl J Med 1984;311: 506.
77. Available at: www.mhakeystonecenter.org. Accessed November 18, 2011.
78. Saint S, Kowalski C, Kaufman S, et al. Preventing hospital-acquired urinary tract infection in the United States: a national study. Clin Infect Dis 2008;46(2):243–50.
79. Dumigan D, Kohan C, Reed C, et al. Utilizing national nosocomial infection surveillance system data to improve urinary tract infection rates in three intensive-care units. Clin Perform Qual Health Care 1998;6(4):172–8.
80. Tucker A, Nembhard I, Edmondson A. Implementing new practices: an empirical study of organizational learning in hospital intensive care units. Manage Sci 2007; 53(6):894–907.

Information Technologies and Patient Safety

Scott J. Ellner, DO, MPH[a,b,]*, Paul W. Joyner, MD[c]

KEYWORDS

• Information • Technology • Surgery • Electronic • Records

The last decade has seen a proliferation of advances in the area of patient safety. At the core of these advances has been the rapid expansion of health information technology (HIT). HIT is defined as the use of electronic and personal health records, automated decision support systems, alerts and reminders, and various technologies for clinical, financial, and administrative purposes.[1,2] HIT has broad applications as an effective tool that can enhance the safety and quality outcomes of the patient across the health care continuum.[3–5]

In 2009, the Health Information Technology for Economic and Clinical Health (HITECH) Act was passed as part of the American Recovery and Reinvestment Act. The Act provided stimulus funding for hospitals and clinicians to implement HIT strategies to improve the quality and safety of patient care.[6] This federally subsidized program authorized the allocation of $27 billion to provide financial incentives for hospitals and clinical practices to adopt and use electronic health information. In addition, HITECH requires the "meaningful use" of electronic health records (EHRs) by eligible providers and hospitals. The core objectives of meaningful use are to improve the delivery of health care. Monetary incentive payments and/or penalties of withholding reimbursement by the Centers for Medicare and Medicaid Services (CMS) will be tied to compliance with the core objectives of meaningful use.[7] The overarching goal, within the provisions of HITECH, is to spur technological advances to improve the health of Americans and the performance of the health care system.[8] The barriers and challenges to universal adoption of an integrated HIT network by health care systems are ever present,[9] but 92% of evidence-based systematic reviews favorably

The authors have nothing to disclose.
^a Department of Surgery, Saint Francis Hospital and Medical Center, 1000 Asylum Avenue, Suite #4320, Hartford, CT 06105, USA
^b University of Connecticut Medical School, Farmington, CT, USA
^c University of Connecticut Residency Program in General Surgery, Department of Surgery, University of Connecticut Health Center, 263 Farmington Avenue, Farmington, CT 06032, USA
* Corresponding author. Department of Surgery, Saint Francis Hospital and Medical Center, 1000 Asylum Avenue, Suite #4320, Hartford, CT 06105.
E-mail address: sellner@stfranciscare.org

Surg Clin N Am 92 (2012) 79–87
doi:10.1016/j.suc.2011.11.002
0039-6109/12/$ – see front matter © 2012 Elsevier Inc. All rights reserved.

surgical.theclinics.com

support its continued development.[10] Increasing acceptance and use of HIT will play a critical role in the enhancement of safety and the quality of care for the surgical patient.

Within the perioperative process, patients are at risk for adverse events from diagnostic and therapeutic errors. The unintended consequence of these errors is the potential harm to the surgical patient. Error prevention and detection strategies using HIT have been advocated to protect patients. A seminal paper by Bates and Gawande[11] described HIT strategies including (1) tools to improve communication, (2) to make knowledge more accessible, (3) to require key pieces of patient information to be available, (4) to perform checks in real time, (5) to assist with monitoring, and (6) to provide support for clinical decision making. Specific applications of these strategies to prevent medication errors have been shown through computerized physician order entry (CPOE),[12] bar code scanning technology,[13] automated tools for safe patient handoffs,[14] surgeon preference cards,[15] and supply inventories. Built-in prompts with alerts and reminders of pending laboratory or radiology results have been shown to facilitate communication for providers.[16]

The operating room provides many opportunities for improvements in patient safety. Innovations in HIT such as bar code technology and radiofrequency identification (RFID) have been applied to creating tracking systems. These technologies have shown promise in decreasing the rate of retained sponges in surgical patients.[17,18] Computerization of perioperative records has facilitated the capture of real-time data to improve documentation and communication by surgeons, anesthesiologists, and operating room personnel.[19,20] An automated operating room computer system designed and based on informatics can provide important data on processes of care and surgical outcomes.[21]

This article describes the current and future framework of HIT as it applies to improvements in safety and quality for the surgical patient through the perioperative process. Specific areas of focus include the use of EHRs to enhance provider communication, intraoperative bar code and RFID technologies for surgical error prevention, informatics to improve operating room situational awareness and team performance, and standardized automated data collection to analyze outcomes.

IMPLEMENTATION OF EHRs FOR SURGICAL CARE

The spectrum of surgical care involves many phases of patient-provider encounters generating a wealth of information. Optimizing the flow of information about the surgical patient within the preoperative, intraoperative, perioperative, and outpatient settings can be challenging. Essential to the successful coordination of care to overcome these challenges are the advances in computerized technology. These advances have provided opportunities to enhance the communication of patient information. The cornerstone of HIT has been the emergence of EHRs providing legible, digitized patient data from various sources within a central, accessible, Web-based repository. Information available within the surgical patient's EHR includes progress notes, operative dictations, CPOE, laboratory and radiological tests, and e-prescribing capabilities. Accessible patient data within an electronic network shared by surgeons, anesthesiologists, subspecialists, nurses, referring providers, and primary care physicians is paramount to the success of the surgical outcome. Whether the patient is a young and healthy individual undergoing a laparoscopic inguinal hernia repair or a complicated, morbidly obese patient requiring an extensive preoperative workup for weight loss surgery, the EHR has the advantage of organizing and providing key information for all providers.

The referral process is an important point of care that can have serious implications for patient outcomes. The communication of patient information from the referring provider to the specialist is essential to a timely and thorough consultation. In addition, the consultative plan from the surgical specialist should be conveyed back to the referring provider to facilitate the transition of care. Studies have shown that an inherent dissatisfaction among primary care providers and specialists exists within the referral process.[22] The reasons for this dissatisfaction include unclear explanation of the patient's active problem, delayed or missing referral reports, and failure by the specialist to respond to the referring provider.[23] The EHR provides a clear synopsis of the patient's problems, facilitates appointment scheduling, and tracks consultative visits. These features have successfully improved communication between providers.[23]

A new generation of computerized health information is a critical adjunct to conveying patient data from the surgeon to the operative team. Through electronic portals, patient information can be transmitted not only to the anesthesiologist but also to the preoperative processing center in a timely fashion to prepare for an upcoming procedure. Key information regarding patient comorbidities, allergies, and active medication use can be electronically communicated to all team members. This procedure allows ample time for the team to review the patient's current health history in collaboration to facilitate the plan of care. A delineated plan of care through a preprocedure briefing, which is understood by the entire team, minimizes the risk of safety-compromising events during the operative procedure.[24,25] Furthermore, a perioperative EHR has been shown to improve throughput and increase efficiency by reducing late case start times and decreasing operating room turnover time.[15]

In the postoperative period, the EHR allows surgeons to update the patient's chart in real time. Important pieces of information such as the type of procedure performed, medication reconciliation, attention to wounds, and dressings can be shared electronically with covering surgeons, the patient's primary caregiver, and nursing and ancillary personnel to prevent adverse outcomes and readmissions. Thirty-day hospital readmissions rates have been reported to occur in 5% to 29% of all medical-surgical inpatient discharges.[26] Inadequate transfer of information regarding patient hospitalizations to transitional care teams has been shown to be an attributable factor to hospital readmissions.[27] Roy and colleagues[28] determined that the results of 41% of inpatient tests were received after discharge. Two-thirds of physicians were unaware of these results, 50% of which required some form of provider intervention.[28] Automated prompts within the EHR alert all providers in the transition of care, facilitating the communication of impending tests or laboratory results that, if missed, could lead to an adverse outcome.

Patients who take an active role in their health care are more likely to experience better outcomes. EHRs have the potential to improve communication between the surgeon and patient. Access to secure portals, interfaced with the EHR system, allows patients, as consumers, to view their medical information.[29,30] This transformative technology empowers patients to view their own personal EHR to share in the decision-making process. Preliminary studies in diabetes management have shown improved outcomes with patient engagement in Web-based portals integrated through EHRs.[31,32] In accordance with stage 1 meaningful use requirements, patients are required to receive a clinical summary of their physician visit within 3 business days.[33] On physician completion of the patient encounter, a clinical summary is automatically generated and delivered for the patient's own personal health record. Most importantly, patients' access to their EHR helps to create trust in the surgeon and fosters informed decision making about the plan of care.

Despite the benefits of EHRs, several limitations and barriers exist to wide-scale adoption. In 2009, only 11.9% of hospitals in the United States had adopted a basic or comprehensive EHR system.[34] Cited barriers include lack of capital for EHR purchase, physician resistance, and inadequacy of hospital staff expertise for maintenance and troubleshooting.[9] For all patients to receive the benefits of EHR, federal policy makers need to address these barriers through improved education, incentives, and technical support.

BAR CODE TECHNOLOGY AND RFID

With the rapid increase in surgical technology, surgeons continue to face challenges for implementation of safe practices for their patients. In the 1999 publication *To Err is Human: Building a Safer Health System* by the Institute of Medicine,[35] it was shown that surgical errors were second only to medication errors as the most frequent cause of error-related deaths. Despite protocols to reduce the potential for error, specifically retained surgical items (RSIs), surgeons as a whole have achieved only limited success. The environment in the operating room is complex with rapid acceleration of newly adapted technology into the surgical field. The operating room staff is faced with an increasing amount of documentation and manual verification in an attempt to decrease RSIs. This requirement can have a measurable impact on operating room efficiency. However, investigation of new technologies to increase efficiency and improve patient safety is now becoming available for implementation.

The occurrence of RSIs continues to be a significant patient safety issue, with approximately 1 occurrence in every 1500 abdominal operations.[36] Every body cavity has been involved in a documented RSI case, but the abdominal cavity continues to be the most common location (46%–55%).[37] Negative outcomes associated with RSI include reoperation, infection, prolonged hospital stays, fistulas, bowel obstruction, and death. In addition, these adverse events erode patient confidence, as well as hospital and practitioner morale. From a financial standpoint, these events are prone to litigation, at times requiring significant payouts to the patient or family, as well as nonreimbursement from the Centers for Medicare and Medicaid Services.

The current standard for all operating centers in the United States requires at least 1 preoperative manual count performed by the surgical technologist and the circulating nurse and at least 1 postoperative count.[38] Many institutions have increased the number of manual counts to include all instruments as well as sponges in an effort to reduce RSIs. As much as 14% of the operating time is spent conducting manual counts.[39] Despite these efforts, studies at large-volume centers have found manual counts to be only 77% accurate.[40] A concern is that some studies have shown that 88% of RSI occurrences were documented to have correct instrument and sponge counts.[41] In an incorrect sponge or instrument count, the recommended practice is to obtain a plain radiograph of the suspected body region. However, even with intraoperative radiographs there has been a failure to detect as many as 33% of RSIs.[40] This highlights that current methods alone are inadequate in the prevention of RSI.

Bar coding and RFID are promising technologies to prevent RSI while enhancing the safety of the surgical patient. Bar coding is ubiquitous in people's daily lives. Bar code technology has become integral in tracking inventory and item identification in nearly every retail point-of-sale system in the United States. Bar coding has also become a popular method for patient identification and medication verification systems in hospitals worldwide.[42,43] The use of bar coded surgical sponges has shown improvements in counting discrepancies compared with traditional counting methods, with a decrease of retained sponges from 12 to 1.7 episodes per 100,000 operations.[41]

RFID is another model currently being evaluated to reduce RSI. This technology, developed in the 1940s, was used by the British military in World War II to identify their aircraft as friendly to antiaircraft batteries.[44] An RFID model has 2 components: a computerized chip containing information and an antenna to receive and transmit information. Placement of implantable chips within surgical sponges has been described for use as part of investigative RFID technology during operative procedures.[45,46] This technology has shown higher sensitivity and specificity compared with surgical counts combined with intraoperative radiographs for identification of retained sponges.[18]

Proprietary sponge accounting and detection systems using bar coding and RFID scanning technology are widely available. These sponge scanning technologies have enormous patient safety implications. In particular, these systems can be used routinely for patients undergoing reoperations after damage control surgery, obesity surgery, and in prolonged operative cases. Moreover, studies have shown that these technologies have empowered nurses to be more confident about speaking up when a sponge count discrepancy exists.[47] The promise of these scanning technologies is encouraging; however, to truly protect the patient from RSI, these technologies must be part of a larger strategy that promotes teamwork and includes the collaboration of the entire surgical team.

Additional uses of RFID technology could potentially be incorporated into real-time monitoring of surgical movements and identification of instruments.[20] This technology is currently being laboratory tested for conceptual use.[48] Through RFID tagging, the location and usage of instrumentation during a procedure could trigger an alert to the surgical team to prepare for changes in the operative plan. For example, uncontrolled, excessive bleeding during laparoscopy would alert the team to the potential for conversion to an open procedure. Prompt notification to the team leaders at the operating room communication desk of a change in plan could generate schedule changes and staff reassignments to maintain optimal workflow. RFID tags in disposable items would allow for continuous monitoring of the operating room inventories, leading to automated orders for purchasing and restocking of supplies.[49]

INTRAOPERATIVE MONITORING AND PATIENT SAFETY

The operating room is a complex environment where critical issues can arise affecting patient safety. Understanding and tracking these issues through computerized intraoperative data systems can help mitigate risk to the patient. Systems are being developed to create a smart operating room that collects data in real time. Automated smart systems would incorporate software to assist in the coordination and completion of not only routine tasks but also those associated with patient safety. For example, the number of circulating nurse room exits is correlated with an increase in patient morbidity.[39] This data collection system would be able to confirm the necessary equipment that is available for the intended procedure, thereby decreasing exits and improving patient safety. Verification of blood products and medication availability can be referenced in real time against a patient's blood type and allergy profile for compatibility.

Communication and coordination are particularly crucial in dynamic environments such as the operating room. One of the largest contributors to errors in surgery has been the lack of communication within the surgical team. Situational awareness is the ability of a team member to identify, process, comprehend, and communicate the crucial elements of information regarding the environment. Variations in the situational awareness of the health care team highlight potential problems related to the specifics of the patient or procedure. This problem is exacerbated by the nature of the operating room in the form of shift changes, breaks, and circulating nurse exits if members of the surgical team are present for only segmented portions of the case. Communication with members of the operating room team with real-time, detailed patient and environmental information facilitates increased efficiency and improved patient safety.[50]

To enhance situational awareness, a black box recorder, similar to those used in the aviation industry, can be used to assess individual and/or team events for quality improvement. Technology like this is needed to collect the complex data to identify and understand the human behaviors that occur in the operating room and their relationship to patient safety events.[50]

AUTOMATED DATA COLLECTION

A highly visible and important issue facing the health care industry is the quality of care provided to patients. To that end, many stakeholders are investing many resources in efforts to collect, analyze, and measure outcomes to improve patient care. Many health care systems use electronic clinical databases to document the care received by patients. Several data collection systems capture information from the patient's medical record to create a platform for outcome measurement and improvement. Data collection systems currently in use include the National Trauma Data Bank, the Society of Thoracic Surgeons (STS) National Database, Cancer Registries, and the American College of Surgeons' National Surgical Quality Program (ACS NSQIP). The preoperative, intraoperative, and postoperative variables collected are based on standardized definitions. These data elements would automatically populate the registry and be available for research. This technology will improve data quality by minimizing the risk of keystroke error during the manual entry of information from medical charts. Automation will also allow the quality team to focus on performance initiatives.

The computerization of data to the registries will provide the seamless transfer of information. Reports generated through automated metrics will guide surgeons, administrators, and operating room teams by supporting clinical decision-making strategies through best practices and evidence-based guidelines.[1] Highly reliable, automated registries are essential to drive performance improvement. As health care reform evolves, regulatory pressures will be ever present and reimbursement will be tied to the accurate measurement of outcomes.

SUMMARY

In the last decade, patient safety has evolved in the discipline of surgery. HIT will play an important role in advancing safety and quality of care for the surgical patient. The electronic health record provides an up-to-date snapshot of important patient information that should be accessible to all health care providers to improve communication. Surgical errors such as retained items can be mitigated through technologies such as bar coding and RFID. Smart operating rooms have the advantage of improving situational awareness to enhance team performance. Automated data registries built with platforms to abstract, analyze, and report back patient outcomes are imperative to drive surgical quality improvement. Surgeons as leaders need to adapt to these advances in HIT. Implementation of health information systems will have a profound effect on optimizing safety and the quality of care provided to patients.

ACKNOWLEDGMENTS

We would like to thank Cynthia Ross-Richardson, MS, BSN, RN, CNOR and Laura Sanzari, BSN, RN for their tireless dedication to the production of this article.

REFERENCES

1. Melton G. Biomedical and health informatics for surgery. Adv Surg 2010;44: 117–30.
2. Evans D, Nichol W, Perlin J. Effect of the implementation of an enterprise-wide electronic health record on productivity in the Veterans Health Administration. Health Econ Policy Law 2006;1(Pt 2):163–9.
3. Doebbeling BN, Vaughn TE, McCoy KD, et al. Informatics implementation in the Veterans Health Administration (VHA) healthcare system to improve quality of care. AMIA Annu Symp Proc 2006;204–8.
4. Fleurant M, Kell R, Love J, et al. Massachusetts e-health project increased physicians' ability to use registries, and signals progress toward better care. Health Aff (Millwood) 2011;30(7):1256–64.
5. El-Kareh R, Gandhi TK, Poon EG, et al. Trends in primary care clinician perceptions of a new electronic health record. J Gen Intern Med 2009;24(4): 464–8.
6. Blumenthal D. Stimulating the adoption of health information technology. N Engl J Med 2009;360(15):1477–9.
7. Blumenthal D, Tavenner M. The "meaningful use" regulation for electronic health records. N Engl J Med 2010;363(6):501–4.
8. Blumenthal D. Launching HITECH. N Engl J Med 2010;362(5):382–5.
9. Jha AK, DesRoches CM, Campbell EG, et al. Use of electronic health records in U.S. hospitals. N Engl J Med 2009;360(16):1628–38.
10. Buntin MB, Burke MF, Hoaglin MC, et al. The benefits of health information technology: a review of the recent literature shows predominantly positive results. Health Aff (Millwood) 2011;30(3):464–71.
11. Bates DW, Gawande AA. Improving safety with information technology. N Engl J Med 2003;348(25):2526–34.
12. Bates DW, Leape LL, Cullen DJ, et al. Effect of computerized physician order entry and a team intervention on prevention of serious medication errors. JAMA 1998;280(15):1311–6.
13. Poon EG, Keohane CA, Yoon CS, et al. Effect of bar-code technology on the safety of medication administration. N Engl J Med 2010;362(18):1698–707.
14. Wayne JD, Tyagi R, Reinhardt G, et al. Simple standardized patient handoff system that increases accuracy and completeness. J Surg Educ 2008;65(6): 476–85.
15. Randa K. Using IT to drive operational efficiency in the OR. Healthc Financ Manage 2010;64(12):90–2, 94.
16. Dalal AK, Poon EG, Karson AS, et al. Lessons learned from implementation of a computerized application for pending tests at hospital discharge. J Hosp Med 2011;6(1):16–21.
17. Greenberg CC, Regenbogen SE, Lipsitz SR, et al. The frequency and significance of discrepancies in the surgical count. Ann Surg 2008;248(2): 337–41.
18. Steelman VM. Sensitivity of detection of radiofrequency surgical sponges: a prospective, cross-over study. Am J Surg 2011;201(2):233–7.
19. Beach MJ, Sions JA. Surviving OR computerization. AORN J 2011;93(2):226–41.

20. Mathias JM. Automation ends preop paper chase. OR Manager 2009;25(6):11–2, 14.
21. Seagull FJ, Moses GR, Park AE. Pillars of a smart, safe operating room. In: Henriksen K, Battles JB, Keyes MA, et al, editors. Advances in patient safety: new directions and alternative approaches (vol. 3: Performance and tools). Rockville (MD): Agency for Healthcare Research and Quality (US); 2008. p. 1–13.
22. Piterman L, Koritsas S. Part I. General practitioner-specialist relationship. Intern Med J 2005;35(7):430–4.
23. Gandhi TK, Keating NL, Ditmore M, et al. Improving referral communication using a referral tool within an electronic medical record. In: Henriksen K, Battles JB, Keyes MA, et al, editors. Advances in patient safety: new directions and alternative approaches (vol. 3: Performance and tools). Rockville (MD): Agency for Healthcare Research and Quality (US); 2008. p. 1–12.
24. Makary MA, Holzmueller CG, Thompson D, et al. Operating room briefings: working on the same page. Jt Comm J Qual Patient Saf 2006;32(6):351–5.
25. Lingard L, Regehr G, Orser B, et al. Evaluation of a preoperative checklist and team briefing among surgeons, nurses, and anesthesiologists to reduce failures in communication. Arch Surg 2008;143(1):12–7 [discussion: 18].
26. Thomas JW, Holloway JJ. Investigating early readmission as an indicator for quality of care studies. Med Care 1991;29(4):377–94.
27. Cummins RO, Smith RW, Inui TS. Communication failure in primary care. Failure of consultants to provide follow-up information. JAMA 1980;243(16):1650–2.
28. Roy CL, Poon EG, Karson AS, et al. Patient safety concerns arising from test results that return after hospital discharge. Ann Intern Med 2005;143(2):121–8.
29. Shaw RJ, Ferranti J. Patient-provider internet portals-patient outcomes and use. Comput Inform Nurs 2011. [Epub ahead of print].
30. Ammenwerth E, Schnell-Inderst P, Hoerbst A. Patient empowerment by electronic health records: first results of a systematic review on the benefit of patient portals. Stud Health Technol Inform 2011;165:63–7.
31. Osborn CY, Mayberry LS, Mulvaney SA, et al. Patient web portals to improve diabetes outcomes: a systematic review. Curr Diab Rep 2010;10(6):422–35.
32. Holbrook A, Thabane L, Keshavjee K, et al. Individualized electronic decision support and reminders to improve diabetes care in the community: COMPETE II randomized trial. CMAJ 2009;181(1–2):37–44.
33. Available at: http://www.cms.gov/EEHRIncentivePrograms/. Accessed July 15, 2011.
34. Jha AK, DesRoches CM, Kralovec PD, et al. A progress report on electronic health records in U.S. hospitals. Health Aff (Millwood) 2010;29(10):1951–7.
35. Kohn LT, Corrigan JM, Donaldson MS. To err is human: building a safer health system. Washington, DC: National Academy Press, Institute of Medicine; 2000.
36. Gawande AA, Studdert DM, Orav EJ, et al. Risk factors for retained instruments and sponges after surgery. N Engl J Med 2003;348(3):229–35.
37. Lincourt AE, Harrell A, Cristiano J, et al. Retained foreign bodies after surgery. J Surg Res 2007;138(2):170–4.
38. Association of Perioperative Registered Nurses (AORN) Recommended Practices Committee. Recommended practices for sponge, sharps, and instrument counts. AORN J 2006;83(2):418, 421–6, 429–33.
39. Christian CK, Gustafson ML, Roth EM, et al. A prospective study of patient safety in the operating room. Surgery 2006;139(2):159–73.
40. Cima RR, Kollengode A, Garnatz J, et al. Incidence and characteristics of potential and actual retained foreign object events in surgical patients. J Am Coll Surg 2008;207(1):80–7.

41. Regenbogen SE, Greenberg CC, Resch SC, et al. Prevention of retained surgical sponges: a decision-analytic model predicting relative cost-effectiveness. Surgery 2009;145(5):527–35.
42. Poon EG, Keohane C, Featherstone E, et al. Impact of barcode medication administration technology on how nurses spend their time on clinical care. AMIA Annu Symp Proc 2006;1065.
43. Nichols JH, Bartholomew C, Brunton M, et al. Reducing medical errors through barcoding at the point of care. Clin Leadersh Manag Rev 2004;18(6):328–34.
44. Landt J. Shrouds of time: the history of RFID. Pittsburgh (PA): Association for Automatic Identification and Mobility; 2001.
45. Macario A, Morris D, Morris S. Initial clinical evaluation of a handheld device for detecting retained surgical gauze sponges using radiofrequency identification technology. Arch Surg 2006;141(7):659–62.
46. Rogers A, Jones E, Oleynikov D. Radio frequency identification (RFID) applied to surgical sponges. Surg Endosc 2007;21(7):1235–7.
47. Mathias JM. Preventing retained items: time to consider technology? OR Manager 2011;27(1):1, 18, 20–2.
48. Kranzfelder M, Schneider A, Blahusch G, et al. Feasibility of opto-electronic surgical instrument identification. Minim Invasive Ther Allied Technol 2009; 18(5):253–8.
49. Shepherd JP, Brickley MR, Jones ML. Automatic identification of surgical and orthodontic instruments. Ann R Coll Surg Engl 1994;76(Suppl 2):59–62.
50. Guerlain S, Adams RB, Turrentine FB, et al. Assessing team performance in the operating room: development and use of a "black-box" recorder and other tools for the intraoperative environment. J Am Coll Surg 2005;200(1):29–37.

Adverse Events: Root Causes and Latent Factors

Richard Karl, MD[a,b,*], Mary Catherine Karl, MBA[a]

KEYWORDS

- Root cause analysis • Theories of error • Systemic factors
- Latent factors

The case was a difficult one. The patient had a large lesion in segments 7 and 8 of her liver: a hepatoma in a setting of hepatitis-C–induced cirrhosis. After careful evaluation, the surgeon recommended resection and the patient agreed. In retrospect, they both might have wished they had not.

The conduct of the case was routine at first. The liver was mobilized; ultrasonography showed no surprises and the blood loss had been minimal. A previous cholecystectomy made the dissection more tedious. Although the procedure took an hour longer than scheduled, the surgeon felt satisfied as she left the resident to close the patient and hurried to clinic.

Postoperatively the patient had a rough course. Fever and increased white blood cell count prompted a computed tomography scan on postoperative day 4. The surgeon felt a chill when she looked at it. There was a lap sponge in the resected bed. Immediate reoperation was proposed and consented. The sponge was densely adherent to the cut surface of the liver and there was significant blood loss. Although the patient was ultimately closed and sent to the intensive care unit, the combination of 10 units of packed red blood cells and underlying liver disease led to a 2-week course of liver failure and then death.

The hospital followed the routine prescribed by the state and the Joint Commission for the Accreditation of Health Care Organizations. The state board of medicine was notified of this sentinel event. Two weeks later a root cause analysis (RCA) was convened by the risk manager. In attendance were the chief safety physician, the chief medical officer, the risk manager, and the vice president in charge of quality and safety. The operating room records, operative notes, and policies for instrument and surgical item counts were reviewed. Interviews had been conducted with the nurses and technicians involved. The surgeon had blamed the resident for the oversight and was generally uncooperative with the investigation. The group decided that 2 errors had occurred: both the scrub and circulating nurse had counted incorrectly. A note was placed in each of their files. The

[a] Department of Surgery, University of South Florida, FL, USA
[b] Surgical Safety Institute, 4951 West Bay Drive, Tampa, FL 33629, USA
* Corresponding author. 12902 Magnolia Drive, FOB-2 Tampa, FL 33612.
E-mail address: rkarl@health.usf.edu

Surg Clin N Am 92 (2012) 89–100
doi:10.1016/j.suc.2011.12.003
0039-6109/12/$ – see front matter © 2012 Elsevier Inc. All rights reserved.

surgeon was reminded of the importance of a thorough examination of the body cavity before closure.

Within a year the nurses involved were brought before the state nurse licensing bureau and reprimanded. The surgeon was fined $10,000 by the state board of medicine for her negligence. The patient's family sued the hospital but not the surgeon or nurses. A settlement was reached. As part of the settlement, both parties agreed not to disclose the terms of the agreement.

A DIFFERENT APPROACH

On December 8, 2005, a Southwest Airlines Boeing 737-700 jet landed at Midway Airport and ran off the end of runway 31C onto Central Avenue, where it struck a car. A child in the car was killed, one occupant sustained major injuries, and 3 others received minor injuries. Eighteen of the 103 occupants of the airplane (98 passengers, 3 flight attendants, and 2 pilots) received minor injuries during the evacuation.

The National Transportation Safety Board (NTSB) convened an investigation that included representatives from Boeing, the engine manufacturers, the avionics manufacturers, the Chicago Aviation Authority, the pilots' and flight attendants' unions, the carrier, the Federal Aviation Administration, and the city of Chicago, among other stakeholders. Two years later the NTSB released its findings.[1] The probable cause was "the pilots' failure to use available reverse thrust in a timely manner to safely slow or stop the airplane after landing, which resulted in a runway overrun." But, the board went on, "This failure occurred because the pilots' first experience and lack of familiarity with the airplane's autobrake system distracted them from thrust reverser usage during the challenging landing."

They did not stop there. Contributing factors were determined:

1. Southwest Airlines' failure to provide its pilots with clear and consistent guidance and training regarding company policies and procedures related to arrival landing distance calculations
2. Southwest Airlines' programming and design of its on-board performance computer
3. Southwest Airlines' plan to implement new autobrake procedures without a familiarization period
4. Southwest Airlines' failure to include a margin of safety in the arrival assessment to account for operational uncertainties
5. The absence of an engineering materials arresting system (at the end of the runway).

LATENT FACTORS AND ROOT CAUSES

These 2 scenarios (1 hypothetical, 1 actual) are emblematic of 2 different philosophies of RCA. In the health care environment, investigations of adverse events are often conducted in secret, with only a few participants. The process frequently concludes that human error was at fault and often recommends remedial training for the persons involved along with some sort of punishment. It is as if the surgeon and the nurses had set a goal to leave a sponge behind in a critically ill patient.

Aviation investigations begin with the premise that the pilots do not want to suffer bodily harm themselves. This premise motivates the investigation in a way that can be readily distinguished from the process in medicine. The NTSB conducts hearings in public and the findings are released to all operators of all similar airplanes. All possible stakeholders participate in the investigation. Several contributing factors are almost always found to be in play in most of the board's investigations.

This article describes the process of RCA, the theories of error that underlie the concept of systemic or latent factors that allow errors to occur or to be propagated without correction; the difference between the process in health care and those found in high-reliability organizations; and suggests some ways to augment the standard health care RCA into a more robust and helpful process.

THEORIES OF ERROR

The widely acknowledged father of human error understanding is James Reason, a British professor of psychology. As early as 1990, Reason was writing about the difference between human error and the systemic conditions that either lead to error or fail to catch and mitigate error. "Aviation is predicated on the assumption that people screw up. You (health care professionals) on the other hand are extensively educated to get it right and so you don't have a culture where you share readily the notion of error. So it is something of a big sea change," he said in an address to the Royal College of Surgeons in 2003.[2]

Reason has categorized two approaches to human error: person and system. In the person approach, most common in health care, the focus is on the people at the sharp end, like the surgeon who leaves a sponge behind. "It views unsafe acts as arising from aberrant mental processes such as forgetfulness, inattention, poor motivation, carelessness, negligence, and recklessness." Solutions to error are naturally enough directed at reducing variability in human behavior. Some time-honored measures include posters that speak to people's sense of fear, writing additional procedures, disciplinary measures, threat of litigation, retraining, naming, blaming, and shaming. Errors are, then, essentially viewed as moral flaws.[3]

The system approach acknowledges that human beings are fallible and that errors are to be expected. Errors are seen as consequences rather than causes, "having their origins not so much in the perversity of human nature as in upstream, systemic factors. Countermeasures include system defenses to prevent or recognize and correct error. When an adverse event occurs, the important issue is not who blundered, but why the defenses failed."[3]

That health care has tended to use the person approach is understandable; it is in line with a tradition of personal accountability, hard work, and diligence: all traits believed to be desirable in health care providers. Reason pointed out that it is more emotionally satisfying and more expedient to blame someone rather than target an institution, its traditions, and power structure (**Table 1**).

Table 1
Reason's person versus system approach

Person Approach	System Approach
Focus on unsafe act of people	Focus on condition of work
Unsafe acts cause error	Upstream systemic factors cause error; human fallibility is unavoidable
Error management by reducing unwanted variability in human behavior	Error management by building system defenses
Uncouple a person's unsafe act from institutional responsibility	Recognize 90% of errors are blameless
Isolate unsafe acts from the system	Remove error-provoking properties of the system
Context-recurrent errors	

Data from Reason J. Human error: models and management. BMJ 2000;320.

However, most human error is unintentional. For instance, in a study of aviation maintenance, 90% of quality lapses were judged blameless.[4,5] This proportion is likely true in all facets of human performance and implies that we spend most of our investigative time on 10% of the problem. Although some small percentage of adverse events are caused by out-of-bounds behavior, most are not. Thus any serious attempt at risk management must take a systems approach: why did this bad thing happen? For this reason, then, a robust investigation into adverse events and near misses to determine the proximate and remote causes is important. Yes, it is true that the Southwest Airlines jet failed to stop on the runway. The real question is why. A search for the root cause becomes a search for the root causes. In another sense, it is not about root; it is about the many factors that can conspire to set up a fertile environment for human error, the last domino, to tip the balance and leave the sponge behind. It is promising that some states, California for example, have begun to fine institutions for sentinel events, not the care provider. It is still a punishment model, but at least the emphasis has shifted to the environment in which the error and subsequent adverse event occurred (**Fig. 1**).

RCA METHODS

Several methodologies exist to assist in guiding a comprehensive, systems-based approach to events, most derived from Reason's system approach to error mentioned earlier. Embracing the conceptual framework (90% of errors are blameless, system issues contribute to most errors, wide sharing of lessons, and so forth) is more important than the specific tool chosen.

Each method presses the participants to think broadly and nonlinearly about the many contributing causes to an error. Only by exploring a comprehensive list of contributing causes can a full list of responsive solutions be developed.

Fishbone

Ishikawa diagrams (also called fishbone diagrams) graphically connect causes with their various effects.[6] Each cause is an opportunity for incremental reduction in the likelihood of the adverse outcome occurring. Causes can be categorized by type such as staff, supervision, material, procedures, communication, environment, or equipment. Categorization brings value in analyzing an aggregation of like events but is less useful in the analysis of an individual event. For instance, it might be useful to know that of the 9 wrong site operations in the last 5 years at the same hospital as the retained sponge case, 60% have been partially caused by team distraction during the time-out. **Fig. 2** is an example of fishbone analysis.

The 5 Whys

Attributed to the Toyota Corporation, the 5 whys urge the analysts to dig deep.

A relentless barrage of "why's" is the best way to prepare your mind to pierce the clouded veil of thinking caused by the status quo. Use it often.

—Shigeo Shingo[7]

Benjamin Franklin's 5-Why Analysis:
For want of a nail a shoe was lost,
for want of a shoe a horse was lost,
for want of a horse a rider was lost,
for want of a rider an army was lost,
for want of an army a battle was lost,
for want of a battle the war was lost,

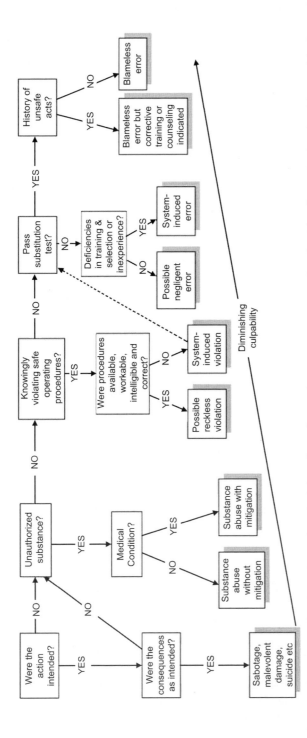

Fig. 1. A decision tree for determining the culpability of unsafe acts. (*From* Reason J. Managing the risks of organizational accidents. Aldershot: Ashgate; 1997. p. 209; with permission.)

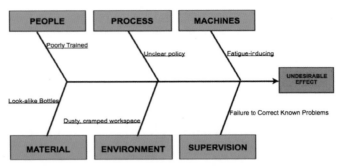

Fig. 2. A fishbone analysis of wrong site operations in a hospital. (*Data from* Ishikawa K. Introduction to quality control. Productivity Press; 1990.)

> *for want of the war the kingdom was lost,*
> *and all for the want of a little horseshoe nail.*[8]

Consider this example. A surgical item was retained. The nurse miscounted. Why? Because he was distracted. Why was he distracted? Because the surgeon was still closing and was asking for more sutures. Why was the count being done before the surgeon had finished closing? And so on. The 5 whys might lead to analyses such as those shown in **Fig. 3**.

These analyses of the miscount are linear. The risk is that they can lead to 1 solution or 1 culprit: the surgeon erred or the nurse erred. One could conclude that there is a magic bullet at the terminus of each example: if that cause were fixed, the offending error would not recur. Be cautious of linear cause maps.

All error derives from complex, at times imperfect, systems. For instance, take the issue of traffic fatalities. Each solution in **Fig. 4** arises from a different cause.[9] Each reduces the likelihood of traffic fatalities. No one solution solely eliminates traffic deaths. Given the inevitability of human error, the risk is never reduced to zero. Highly safe systems layer on error-avoiding and error-trapping processes to reach their acceptable level of risk. The more defenses, the lower the risk of error occurring and not being caught. The cost of each intervention can be evaluated in relationship to the cost of human lives.

Reason's Swiss cheese diagram (**Fig. 5**) shows several levels of defenses against inevitable human error. **Fig. 5** is an example of Reason's multilayered approach to error as adapted to the surgical environment.

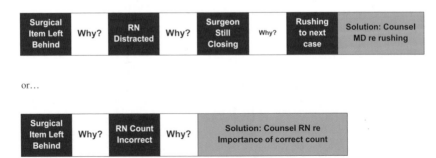

Fig. 3. An example of the 5 whys. RN, registered nurse.

Seat Belts
Reduced speed limits
Crush Bumpers
Greater police presence
Risk
Effectiveness of Solutions

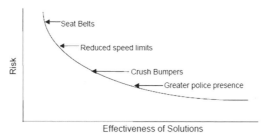

Fig. 4. Risk versus effectiveness of solutions. (*Courtesy of* M. Galley.)

MULTIPLE CAUSES ANALYSIS

Let's rethink the earlier retained surgical item (RSI) scenario. The nurse miscounted. Why? Because he was distracted *and* the odds of a count of 100 items being in error is $\pm 10\%$. Why was he distracted? Because the music was loud, the beepers were going off, the surgeon had not closed and was asking for more sutures during the count, and there was mental pressure to get the next case started. If we built a graph of this cause analysis it would be multipronged and complex. It would represent the many system issues that bear on the outcome. Each cause would have its own effects and its own possible solutions: a more robust and fruitful analysis. An example is given in **Fig. 6**.

This way of thinking leads to a distinction between the term root cause (singular,) connoting one, primary, dominate cause, and an alternate approach that analyzes many possible causes (plural). Although the NTSB does conclude with one probable cause, it also goes on to list many contributing causes for each accident.

An alternate approach dispenses with prioritization of causes. Causes have corresponding solutions so the objective is to discover all causes and the resultant array of solutions. In this approach the solutions, not the causes, are prioritized as to their ease, cost of implementation, and effectiveness. The multicause approach supports

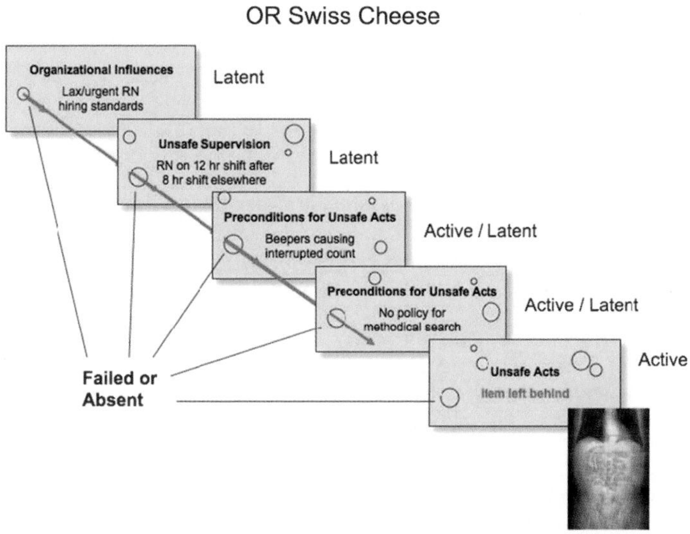

OR Swiss Cheese
Organizational Influences
Lax/urgent RN hiring standards
Latent
Unsafe Supervision
RN on 12 hr shift after 8 hr shift elsewhere
Latent
Preconditions for Unsafe Acts
Beepers causing interrupted count
Active / Latent
Preconditions for Unsafe Acts
No policy for methodical search
Active / Latent
Unsafe Acts
Item left behind
Active
Failed or Absent

Fig. 5. Operating room Swiss cheese model. RN, registered nurse. (*Data from* Reason J. Human error: models and management. Br Med J 2000; 320.)

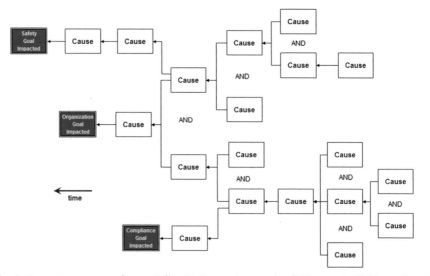

Fig. 6. A root cause map. (*From* Galley M. Improving on the fishbone. Available at: http://www.thinkreliability.com/Root-Cause-Analysis-Articles.aspx. Accessed August 29, 2011; with permission.)

Reason's system versus person approach to error and recognizes the latent conditions that lead to, support, and may create error.

Continuing with the RSI example, a multipronged cause analysis would arrive at several solutions, each of which would reduce (but not eliminate) the risk of RSI. Some possibilities include:

1. Assertive reduction and management of the environmental distractions such as pagers, music and door openings.
2. A required search of the body cavity by both the Attending and the Resident.
3. Clarity that ensuring the extant case goes well outweighs any institutional pressure to start the next case (along with a change in the policies that might provide the pressure).
4. A high tech wand detection system to perform a final check for RSIs.
5. Mandatory radiographs in cases in which the count is unreconciled.

Each of these solutions can be evaluated and prioritized based on their ability to reduce the risk of RSI and their total cost. Considering Reason's Swiss cheese model, several of the possible error-reducing or error-catching tools may be layered into the process, depending on the level of risk the hospital is willing to take.

Many people think of cause and effect as a linear relationship, where an effect has a cause. In fact, cause-and-effect relationships connect based on the principle of a system. A system has parts just like an effect has causes...Most organizations mistakenly believe that an investigation is about finding the 1 cause–or a "root cause."[9]

A further advantage of the multicause approach to analysis and resolution is that the chosen corrections flow directly from the causes. Solutions imposed on the organization that obviously bear little relationship to what the staff know to be the issues lead to disparagement of the RCA process. Worse yet, a barrage of solutions unrelated to the underlying causes is thrown at the organization, potentially further deteriorating the work environment with extra steps and procedures not related to the discovered causes.

THE CONSEQUENCES OF THE PERSON APPROACH TO MEDICAL ERROR

In September, 2010, Kimberly Hiatt, a critical care nurse in Seattle Children's Hospital, made a medication error that contributed to the death of an 8-month-old child. She was fired by the hospital and investigated by the state's nursing commission. In April 2011, she killed herself.[10] This terrible consequence shows the price we pay as a profession for the secrecy and judgmental approach to medical error. In medication errors, root cause analyses frequently find several systemic causes, like the similarity in appearance of bottles with different dosages; arithmetical errors in situations in which no double-check system is in place; fatigue; and inadequate hand-off policies.

It is estimated that 250 doctors commit suicide yearly, a rate about twice that of the general population. For those involved in medical error, the rate of contemplating suicide is three times higher than other physicians. The sense of responsibility for and chagrin about a mistake weighs heavily on our fellow caregivers.[11]

SECRECY, MALPRACTICE, AND ERROR

Some risk managers in US hospitals may tell you that their job is to keep the institution out of trouble and out of the newspapers. Fear of litigation and public exposure is a cultural hallmark of medicine. This situation is in direct contradiction of the principle of widely shared error, open exploration of the causes of adverse events, and a just culture. These barriers to cause analysis are described in detail elsewhere in this issue.

DO RCAs WORK?

Recently concern has been voiced about the usefulness of RCAs in health care. Why is it that a tool used so effectively by the NTSB has not become commonplace and useful in medicine? Wu and colleagues[12] noted that many medical RCAs were conducted incompletely or incorrectly. These investigators found that many placed inappropriate emphasis on finding the single most common reason. Furthermore, implementing actions in response to RCA findings, even modest ones, was difficult. Politics, resources, and lack of understanding of the RCA process were attributed causes for several instances in which the hospital had repeated adverse events of the same nature even after several obvious causes had been uncovered in RCA. This finding leads some administrators to discount the process as unhelpful. Adding to that concern is the worry that RCA content is discoverable during malpractice litigation further reinforces the blame, secrecy, and self-protective political environment that may make another event occur.

A UK study by Nicolini and colleagues[13] suggests that RCAs are prone to inconsistent application and misuse. Management can use the process to increase governance hegemony, and those on the investigation side of the process have many clever ways to subvert the intent of the RCA, especially when their expertise, motivation, or sincerity is called into question. These investigators conclude that a "failure to understand the inner contradictions, together with unreflective policy interventions, may produce counterintuitive negative effects which hamper, instead of further, the cause of patient safety"

It seems obvious that without a national overseeing body such as the Federal Aviation Administration and the NTSB, RCAs carried out in one hospital, no matter how excellent and telling, are not likely to be of use in neighboring institutions.

SCENARIO 1: ULTIMATE RESOLUTION

In the case of the liver resection described at the beginning of this article, a new physician safety officer was appointed and charged with revisiting the RSI. This time the RCA was carried out to attempt to find the underlying causes and contributing factors leading to the adverse event.

The RCA was convened at noon on a Wednesday. The chief operating officer of the hospital, the chief financial officer, the chairwoman of the surgery department, the chair of anesthesiology, and the nursing director of the operating room were all present. In addition, the hospital had invited a representative of the patient's family to participate. The nurses, technicians, surgeons, and residents involved in the case were all present. The timing, the location, and the attendees all signaled interest in this process at the highest levels of the organization.

The findings were revealing. The surgeon, pressured to be in clinic after the operation, had left a resident to close. There were metrics in place to dissuade the surgeon from being late to clinic; and there was no mechanism by which a surgeon could have a valid priority reason to be tardy. The resident was new; he had never worked with this surgeon before and had assumed that the surgeon had performed an extensive body cavity search for RSIs. The hospital did not have any policy regarding responsibility of the surgical team for cavity searches. For that matter, the hospital had never specified who was responsible for closing any surgical patient's wound.

Interviews with the nursing staff were also illuminating. During the closing first count, the circulating nurse was relieved for lunch in the middle of the count. The new nurse did not restart the count, but picked up where the previous nurse had left. Examination of the operating room computer system found that the first and second counts were marked as correct by the relieving circulator. A literature search concluded that the chance of a counting error was 10 in 100, making reliance on counting procedures alone unlikely to achieve the goal of no retained items. The resident testified that he felt hurried; the attending expected him in clinic as soon as possible. He acknowledged that he directed that the radio be turned up loud so that he could hear some rock and roll.

Interviews with the patient's family were troublesome. The patient complained of an unusual, and new, back pain immediately after surgery. The family was puzzled also by her complaint of right shoulder pain. The family expressed frustration that these complaints were met with a patronizing attitude by both nurses and physicians attending the patient. When finally told of the retained surgical item, the patient had said, "I knew something was bad wrong."

In the end, the RCA group concluded their work with a report not dissimilar to the NTSB report cited earlier. They found that the probable cause of the retained sponge, reoperation, and subsequent death was distraction of the operating room personnel at the time the sponges were counted. Contributing factors were:

1. Failure to perform a careful body cavity search
2. No clear hospital policy regarding cavity search requirements by the operative team
3. No policy for distracting music, beepers, or phone calls in surgical suites
4. No guidelines for the responsibility of the attending surgeon to be present for the entire operation
5. Unworkable attendance requirements for clinic attendance that had the effect of distracting caregivers in other parts of the hospital
6. Lack of consistent application of existing policies already in place regarding time-outs, pre operative and postoperative briefings, which led to inconsistent conduct of these tools

7. Lack of policy prohibiting team member relief during high-stress portions of the procedure (the team noted that the peak stress period was different for the nursing team, anesthesia team, and the surgical team).

The new chief executive officer (CEO) of the hospital received the report and posted it on internal and external Web sites. She directed the chairs of surgery and anesthesia and the director of nursing to convene a group of in-house experts to develop workable policies that would address the issues discovered. Policies for relief, time-outs, briefings, counts, and distractions were developed. The hospital CEO directed that repetitive outlying behavior by any member of staff be directed to her exclusively. Additional staff was hired to manage beepers and phone calls during surgery. A team of physicians without operative responsibilities was appointed to deal with inpatient and outpatient issues while the operative team was in the operating room. All solutions flowed logically and directly from the causes identified in and disclosed from the RCA so that they made operational sense to the individuals performing the work. The new way of doing things was believed to be home grown, not enforced from the top.

When queried by a reporter at an event honoring the hospital as the safest in the nation, the CEO said, "I had no idea as to the chaotic environment in which we used to ask our hard working, altruistic people to work. I didn't accomplish this, they did. They did an analysis of each problem that was robust, non-linear, thoughtful and not judgmental. Then they came to our administrative team and proposed changes. Since many of the administrators, including me, had been at the RCA and heard the patient's family speak, they had no trouble convincing us to apply the resources and the support, both administratively and emotionally, for a safe environment. It is the people on the front lines that know what needs to be done."

WHEN TO PERFORM CAUSE ANALYSIS

Are cause analyses performed only for major sentinel events? Commercial aviation found its major events occurring so infrequently that to continue to improve, it had to focus on daily system imperfections. It developed a robust, nonjeopardy near-miss reporting system to gather those imperfections. Cause analyses should be performed on aggregated events because sentinel events occur infrequently. Cause analysis can be performed for any process error even if it did not produce an unfavorable outcome. Only when health care develops a serious system for tracking and acting on near misses will patient safety improve.

REFERENCES

1. Runway Overrun and Collision Southwest Airlines Flight 1248 Boeing 737-7H4, N471WN Chicago Midway International Airport Chicago, Illinois December 8, 2005. Accident Report. National Transportation Safety Board AAR-07/06. Available at: http://www.ntsb.gov/doclib/reports/2007/AAR0706.pdf. Accessed June 29, 2011.
2. Reason J. Problems and perils of prescription medicine. London: Royal College of Physicians; 2003.
3. Reason J. Human error: models and management. Br Med J 2000;320:768–70.
4. Marx D. Discipline: the role of rule violations. Ground Effects 1997;2:1–4. Available at: http://www.system-safety.com/articles/GroundEffects/Volume%202%20Issue%204.pdf. Accessed December 14, 2011.

5. Reason J. Managing the risks of organizational accidents. Aldershot (UK): Ashgate; 1997.
6. Ishikawa K. Introduction to quality control. London: Productivity Press; 1990.
7. Available at: http://matthrivnak.com/lean-quotes. Accessed January 3, 2012.
8. Available at: http://www.moresteam.com/toolbox/5-why-analysis.cfm. Accessed January 3, 2012.
9. Galley M. Improving on the fishbone. Available at: http://www.thinkreliability.com/Root-Cause-Analysis-Articles.aspx. Accessed August 29, 2011.
10. Nurse's suicide highlights twin tragedies of medical errors: Kimberly Hiatt killed herself after overdosing a baby, revealing the anguish of caregivers who make mistakes. JoNel Aleccia; 2011. Available at: http://msnbc.com. Accessed August 29, 2011.
11. O'Reilly K. Revealing their medical errors; why three doctors went public 2011. Available at: http://amednews.com. Accessed August 29, 2011.
12. Wu A, Lipshuts A, Provonost P. Effectiveness and efficiency of root cause analysis in medicine. JAMA 2009;299:685–7.
13. Nicolini D, Waring J, Mengis J. Policy and practice in the use of root cause analysis to investigate clinical adverse events: mind the gap. Soc Sci Med 2011;73: 217–22.

Making Sense of Root Cause Analysis Investigations of Surgery-Related Adverse Events

Bryce R. Cassin, RN, AFCHSM[a,b,*], Paul R. Barach, MD, MPH[c,d]

KEYWORDS

- Root cause analysis • Patient safety • Adverse events
- Sense making • Structured conversation

> May it not be that our naïve intuitions are not so far wrong after all and that causal laws in relation to persons are few because persons are not entirely subject to them.[1]

WHAT HAS BEEN LEARNED FROM ROOT CAUSE ANALYSIS ABOUT SURGERY-RELATED ADVERSE EVENTS?

The conversation related to patient safety has gained currency in the last decade and incident investigation processes have been implemented by health care organizations internationally to improve the safety of clinical care delivery.[2] The most common method used as a primary means of investigating serious adverse events is root cause analysis (RCA).[3] The Institute of Medicine's (IOM) report, *To Err is Human*, stated that "root causes are complicated by the fact that several interlocking factors often contribute to an error or series of errors that in turn result in an adverse event."[4] Two significant facts emerge from this quotation: the IOM investigators view error as causally linked to medical management (or rather, bad systems) and that the complication they describe is one of collecting administrative data for the purpose of raising awareness of the issues, not taking specific action to better understand

[a] University of Western Sydney, School of Nursing and Midwifery, Locked Bag 1797, Penrith South DC, New South Wales 1797, Australia
[b] University of Technology, School of the Built Environment, PO Box 123 Broadway, Sydney, New South Wales 2007, Australia
[c] Utrecht Medical Centre, University of Utrecht, PO Box 85500, GA 3508 Utrecht, Netherlands
[d] University of Stavanger, 4036 Norway
* Corresponding author. University of Western Sydney, School of Nursing and Midwifery, Locked Bag 1797, Penrith South DC, New South Wales 1797, Australia.
E-mail address: bryce.cassin@gmail.com

Surg Clin N Am 92 (2012) 101–115
doi:10.1016/j.suc.2011.12.008
0039-6109/12/$ – see front matter © 2012 Elsevier Inc. All rights reserved.

surgical.theclinics.com

the clinical workplace.[2] The IOM report was primarily concerned with presenting hard numbers to draw public attention to patient safety.[2] The chosen vehicle at the time was error counting and reporting systems. Making sense of the situations behind the interlocking factors and bad systems is now more important than a statistical count of errors, a retrospective search for causes, or high-level planning documents about top-down system redesign.[5] Key advocates in the patient safety movement acknowledge that current systems are too complex to expect people to perform perfectly all of the time and that leaders have to put in place systems that support safe practice.[2]

There is an urgent need to build ground-up capacity to make sense of the complexity in care systems having raised awareness about improving patient safety. The next stages in the patient safety movement's plan must involve practical experimentation with meaningful tools and methods at the local level where clinical teams can own and control improvement not as a time-limited administrative project, but as a natural part of the ongoing shaping of habits and routines in care delivery. For example, to better understand the clinical context of complex care, significant investment is being made in surgical simulation and skills development.[6] After more than a decade of significant investment in improvement activities such as RCA, it is timely that due consideration is given to assessing the quality of information available and how it is interpreted, because many myths prevail.

Has progress been made in better understanding the interlocking factors in the clinical work environment by collecting data? There is a pervasive belief among advocates of the patient safety movement that all errors in a health system are discoverable and preventable. Senior industry leaders involved in the 1999 IOM Report have pushed toward achieving zero incidence of errors, and more and better data[2]; it is not an isolated view.[7,8] The belief is primarily that having more information is sufficient to improve health systems. However, there is no palpable sense in administrative data of the reality of delivering care in unpredictable situations. The more sensitive analyses based on expertise in accident investigation acknowledge that "adverse events should be characterized as emergent properties of complex systems; they cannot be predicted."[9] Perhaps the explanatory hypotheses for getting, doing, and talking about bad systems need revision to make better observations of clinical care.[1] Many errors are preventable and, through the RCA process, system flaws are identified, recommendations are made, and sometimes solutions are implemented, only to see the problem recur. Simple equipment failures can be addressed via high-level system responses that replace or fix the broken part, but many RCAs relate to complex social, emerging interaction issues that require action at multiple levels of the system, from the local clinical unit, to teams, departments, and whole facilities. If RCA is only suited to a high-level analysis of specific, prevalent problems,[10] why is it still extensively used across health systems to investigate all types of serious adverse events?

This article draws on the experience of facilitating more than 100 RCA investigations across one Australian health delivery service in New South Wales. Several themes emerged from reviewing these RCAs that are relevant in understanding the surgical context. These themes (**Table 1**) represent a mixture of the outcomes of clinical care (eg, procedural complications) and explanations relating to problems in the clinical environment (eg, skill mix of the surgical team, and missed diagnoses). The purpose in reviewing the surgery-related RCAs here is not to attempt a comprehensive classification system but to highlight the patterns that emerge from the RCA reports that may assist clinical leaders in determining priorities in relation to improvement activities. The number of themes and issues carries no predictive value, nor are they characterized as causal to the outcomes of the events. Their significance is in their descriptive value of RCAs and as design challenges relative to particular situations in the clinical workplace.

Table 1 Themes and issues identified from surgery-related RCAs	
Theme	Issues Identified
Failure to recognize or respond appropriately to the deteriorating patient within the required timeframe	Post-CABG complications Postoperative sepsis Postoperative hyponatremia
Workforce availability and skills	Orientation, training, and supervision of new or junior members of the surgical team, especially outside normal working hours
Transfer of patients for surgery	Difficulty in organizing an OR for surgery Failure to hand over information about patient acuity
The management of trauma	Coordination and response of trauma teams Clinical decision-making process for patients with trauma Coordination of care between multiple clinicians
Access to emergency OR	Antepartum hemorrhage and emergency cesarean Urgent orthopedic procedure Urologic complications requiring urgent surgery
Missed diagnosis	Thoracolumbar fracture in a patient with trauma Brain abscess mistaken for cerebral metastasis Subarachnoid hemorrhage thought to be drug overdose
Unexpected procedural complications	Airway obstruction after thyroidectomy Failed intubation
Sentinel events	Wrong site procedure: spinal fusion at wrong level Retained surgical products requiring surgical removal

Abbreviation: OR, operating room.
Data from The analysis is derived from a metropolitan health service, Sydney, NSW, Australia. Personal communication, Deputy Director for Clinical Governance, January 2007.

A visual survey of **Table 1** shows that it is difficult to draw generalizations from RCA data because the issues are multifactorial and require a systemic response. The data are presented as they were reported to show that making sense of the themes and issues requires further information about the RCAs. We draw attention to the importance of assessing RCA data in context to gain a meaningful understanding of the clinical workplace. Our RCA data may or may not inform the clinical risk management processes in other surgical centers. The themes mentioned are likely to be familiar, but so too is the experience of frustration with the quality of detailed information emerging from the RCA reports. Citing these themes and issues arising from RCA reports illustrates the complex nature of the problems involved. The formal RCA process seeks out clearly identified problems, where facts can be analyzed, efficient solutions recommended and effectively implemented, and the system of care modified quickly and rationally. However, the problems cited are never simple or easy (see **Table 1**). These complex problem situations have been identified as so-called wicked problems that are characteristic because they resist easy formulation, cannot be easily isolated from the system of care, have no clear causal relationship, are not exhaustive descriptions of the problem, and can be explained in many ways.[11] Wicked problems are related to other problems, have no simple fix, but require a specific response that only makes sense in the context of the unique characteristics attached to the problem described. What is missing from **Table 1** is the real-world settings of the problems, and how clinicians at the time of the events concerned made sense of the situation that confronted them, with its unpredictable and contingent characteristics.

WHAT HAS BEEN LEARNED FROM RCA?

A central hypothesis proposed by the article is that the environment of clinical practice and the thinking it entails resist reduction to stable and standardized risk identification. First, the historical context of the everyday experiences of clinicians is not captured by statistical measures used in evidence-based medicine. Second, the clinical experience is more dynamic than the simple cause-and-effect sequences constructed in RCA flow charts and investigations. This problematic situation warrants open and frank discussion to identify a more effective model of inquiry.

A key observation that emerged from the experience of facilitating multiple RCAs is that the methodology has a limited usefulness beyond sequencing facts and listing problems.[12] There is a tendency among clinicians to focus thinking around familiar evidence-based clinical models in which statistical variation in clinical medicine can be measured and the probability of its significance quantified.[13] However, understanding the dynamic interaction and communication problems that arise from the social complexity of clinical work, the most common issues identified by RCA, is not a subset of clinical medicine. Developing an understanding of unexpected events in the clinical setting requires a different set of tools and mental model. The clinical workplace is not a controlled experimental environment and its risks are ambiguous, constantly emerging, and unpredictable. Risks in clinical care delivery are situational and context specific. The clinical workplace needs to be understood in its temporal context, where managing constraints and negotiating the boundaries of safe practice is a matter of collective expertise and experience. This context requires reflection on clinical judgment and decision making. When RCA teams are faced with the complexity of a past event, there is no experimental control, nor any assurance that their recommended actions will reduce the risk of recurrence of the event in the future.

Public and political interest in the outcomes of RCA has shifted the focus of attention from the context-specific nature of the situations investigated by RCA to the collection of abstract categories of information that satisfy the need for generalized administrative data. The continuous flow of activity in the clinical workplace cannot be reduced to simple data mining and dredging. What is significant in one event, with its unique set of circumstances and mix of clinical expertise and environmental factors, is unlikely to be true or applicable to another event simply because it is given a similar label in administrative data sets.

Surgery-related adverse events rarely present as discrete causal sequences within the clinical setting. RCA teams respond pragmatically in team meetings by reflecting on broader issues in the clinical workplace drawing on their own experience and observations, which raises questions about the limitations of RCA as a key method of analysis and the compensatory role of the expertise of RCA teams, including:

1. Why have RCAs failed to significantly improve the capability (ie, safety, quality, reliability) of care delivery systems?
2. How do RCA teams compensate for the limitations of the RCA methodology?
3. What can be learned from accident analysis models about the alternatives to RCA?

MEASURING SAFETY: THE ACCIDENT PARADOX

Many organizations use RCA-driven adverse event data as an index of the relative safety of their constituent parts or subsystems. Adverse events, like the number of errors, are poor indicators of the general safety of the system.[14] Only if the system has complete control over the factors causing adverse events and near misses could an adverse event history provide a reliable measure of its safety. Hazards can be moderated but they cannot be eliminated, which may lead to the accident paradox in which safe organizations can still have bad adverse events, whereas unsafe systems can escape them for long periods. Furthermore, progress creates new risk that is difficult to anticipate but is a feature of new procedures and technologies.[15]

One way to resolve this paradox is to recognize that safety has two aspects. The positive aspect of safety (ie, intrinsic resistance to chance combinations of hazards, unsafe acts, technical failures), like good health, is difficult to define and even harder to measure. By comparison, the absence of safety, like poor health, is clearly signaled by near misses, injuries, and fatalities, which lend themselves to close analysis and quantification. However, the data provided by RCA accident and incident reporting systems, although essential for understanding the causes of past mishaps, are both too little and too late to support measures directed at enhancing a system's intrinsic safety.[16]

Many organizations treat safety management like a negative production process. They assess their negative RCA outcome data and then set themselves reduced targets for the coming accounting period. The trouble with this approach is that errors and adverse events are not directly manageable. A more effective model for safety management is to monitor the system's process or vital signs on a regular basis (ie, indices relating to quality management, equipment design, workplace design, conditions of work, safety procedures, communications, maintenance, and so on) like a long-term fitness program. The program is designed to help clinicians and managers bring about continuous, step-by-step improvement in the system's intrinsic resistance to chance combinations of latent failures, human fallibility, and hazards. This program entails managing the manageable: that is, the organizational human factors that lie within the direct spheres of influence of clinicians as they go about their daily work.[17]

In contrast with a systematic approach to continuous improvement,[18] the introduction of mandated RCA investigations for serious adverse events requires clinicians and managers to isolate elements in the workplace systems for attention without reference to the other parts of the system. Health service managers and policy makers invest considerable resources and commitment in RCA educational programs because they assure a degree of control and certitude in managing the clinical environment. RCA promises greater control over clinical practice through the identification of corrective actions, but with no clear process for implementation of, nor accountability over, the recommended changes. Tangible benefits to the clinical setting are needed to achieve clinician buy-in. Strong murmurs of discontent and cynicism were initially observed (for medical staff, RCAs were only a small part of a bigger problem to do with a general lack of an overarching view of the system).[19] RCA meetings also created an opportunity for improved communication in the workplace through organized sense making, which was otherwise ad hoc. This opportunity entailed a process whereby different approaches to noticing and bracketing clinical care are shared across the boundaries of specialism, expertise, and different clinical disciplines.[20]

HAVE RCAs ALTERED THE IMPROVEMENT CAPABILITY OF SURGICAL CENTERS?

The emphasis in RCAs on causation and error management is not an effective method to engage clinicians nor to improve understanding of the clinical workplace. Perhaps the wrong questions have been asked about adverse events by focusing on categorizing error and crafting causation statements rather than asking how clinicians maintain their continuity of practice amidst the changing and dynamic conditions that characterize the clinical work environment.

The RCA process has recently been defined as an essential tool of vigorous system investigation, assessment, learning, and improvement, with an emphasis on respectful engagement of frontline clinical staff, patients, and families in the process.[21] This shift is an important step forward by recognizing the important role of the *conversation space* in RCA investigations. Previously, the focus in RCA programs has been on the stepwise process of causal reasoning.[3] Changing the focus to capture the agency of the people involved will enable institutional assumptions in the RCA process to be questioned around:

1. Do disruptions to clinical practice ever happen in sequence?
2. Are problems, once fixed, less likely to recur?
3. Are root causes quantifiable for particular events as categorized in reports?

These goals have more to do with the mission of government and large agencies around comparable performance measurement than improving health care outcomes. RCA reports omit the significant detail that surgical microsystems need to know to improve the safety of their local practice. The context relates to specific times, and places for patients, clinicians, and managers interacting around care delivery in constantly changing and often uncertain circumstances. Government policy assumes that information gathered from RCA reports will translate into corrective actions but without an identifiable process for implementing practical change nor due regard for the differences between local clinical contexts. Lee Clarke,[22] an organizational sociologist, describes concentrated managerial initiatives like RCA as a rational process to tame risk and uncertainty, opining that:

> When organizations analyze problems, they try to transform uncertainties into risks, rationalizing problems previously outside the realm of systematic control... The organizational urge behind these transformations is part of the characteristic drive for rationalization in modern society... this urge reflects a societal-level expectation that organizations should be able to control the uncertain, and be able to respond effectively to the untoward.[22]

The belief that there are causes to be discovered in the organization is socially constructed from the benefit of hindsight after an event.[23] We observed that working with people in the visceral setting of the RCA team meeting was a more meaningful way of capturing the collective mindset as people discussed how flexible and adaptable strategies were routinely used, including workarounds and variations from local policies. This normalized deviance in which workarounds and rule breaking were part of everyday work caused surprise at times to risk management personnel, but, for clinical personnel, was seen as part of getting the job done. Surgical microsystems require something more than rational planning when responding to unexpected events. There is a risk that RCA reports only hold symbolic value at a policy and senior management level. The proliferation of collated reports about RCA findings provides no traction for making sense of the local complexity in surgical work environments.

Public reporting on RCA outcomes dilutes the rich contextual information clinicians need to respond to problematic situations in the clinical workplace. The multiple layers of bureaucratization that prevent timely feedback on RCA findings have increasingly frustrated clinicians and led to delays in immediate attention to the system solutions that could be implemented. Monitoring RCA report outcomes has morphed over time into a sustainable specialism within health departments. Multiple systems for gathering event data have been developed, reducing comparability, rendering the possibility of system level learning even less feasible. The statutory and professional requirements for mandatory reporting (eg, deaths in surgery, deaths under anesthesia, and medico-legal claims) have generated databases for these types of events and resulted in more predictable event reporting (eg, there is widespread focus on identification of the deteriorating patient, preventing wrong-sided surgery, improving clinical handover, and increasing hand washing among clinicians). As reporting systems multiply, it is imperative that effective structures are put in place at the hospital level where organizational factors associated with clinical adverse events are best understood.

Drilling down to the level of specific incident types and the practice of listing and categorizing events is not sensitive to the changing nature of serious risks in different contexts within and across health services. RCAs reveal considerable variation in the way adverse events are perceived by different clinicians and clinical teams. High-level descriptive analyses of RCAs may be able to highlight local patterns but rational-looking labels in collated reports of adverse events do not improve the ability of local clinicians to manage the constraints in their particular clinical environment. What fascinates RCA teams and occupies the local clinical review meetings is how problems emerge and how best to respond to messy situations and breakdowns in safety. RCA teams and local clinicians need to understand the connections between people at an individual, team, department, and interdepartment and cross-team level.[24] RCA teams are particularly good at looking at small pieces of problems and grasping the complexity that exists across their hospital or health service. The solutions that emerge from RCA team discussions respond to the specific embedded routines and habits of local clinical teams. Their concern is not with causes, but shedding light in a manner that makes sense to the people who will need to adapt their practices in response to the next unexpected event: "if such things can somehow be made visible, a fuller range of counter measure becomes available beyond telling frontline operators to be more careful."[25]

It is noteworthy that only a small number of sociotechnical events have identifiable causes, because most adverse events involve complex social and cultural problems.[26,27] Failure at a bureaucratic level to grasp the importance of local clinical perceptions and sense making limits the usefulness of RCA as a tool for improvement in health services. Although concrete actions recommended in RCA reports have been successfully implemented for stable technology and equipment-related issues (eg, bar code technology for medication administration, electronic medical record systems), it has been harder for large patient-safety agencies to grasp communication with frontline clinical staff as a source of organizational intelligence, beyond compliance with administrative reporting systems.[28]

Moving the discussion closer to the mindset of physicians and surgeons reveals another problem: a widespread assumption that understanding adverse events is a subset of logical clinical care. Senior clinicians contributing to RCA teams look for elements within events where means and ends can be identified and cause-and-effect thinking has rational application (such as the interpretation of a clinical event using case-based reasoning).[29] The combined impact of promoting causal reasoning in RCA investigations and defaulting to a search for clinical causes is to give the impression of an explanation of complex social and cultural problems in adverse events, when instead these issues require an approach to inquiry that can shed light on particular clinical environments.[30] This kind of thinking is more like the practical judgment and decision making surgeons apply in the operating room where patient circumstances are unpredictable and information is incomplete. A surgical team assesses situations by surveying and evaluating the work environment, where they consciously identify what is new or different, not by looking for causes or stable qualities via some abstract notion of a health care system.[31]

At the heart of understanding an adverse event is a realization of the pragmatic thinking skills of clinical assessment that help create an awareness of situations. RCA team members apply the same attentional and perceptual skills to interpret an adverse event as they would an altered situation in the surgical intensive care unit, in the absence of any meaningful access to what made sense to their peers at the time of the past event under review. RCA teams function like clinicians in the workplace who manage real situations where expertise, workload, and expectations are highly variable factors.[31] However, the value of practical clinical reasoning is lost in the causal language of RCA talk. RCA documents make claims that strive to reduce uncertainty, whereas clinicians have learned to live with it and embrace its richness.

The specific causes of an event are not discoverable; there is no root or primary cause that can be identified as an end point because the workflow in an organization is continuous.[25,27] The RCA training material asks RCA teams to look for the sources of error in the system of care but does not equip RCA teams, beyond a rudimentary introduction to human factors concepts, with the detailed cognitive human factors training to make practical recommendations that address the system complexity.[32]

The simplified list of human factors categories in the US Veterans Administration (VA) National Center for Patient Safety (NCPS) RCA triage card (**Table 2**) can be likened to a 'constant accident model' (**Fig. 1**) in which the thinking about adverse events is not discreet, but oscillates between technical and equipment causes, issues in relation to human performance, and factors within the organization.[12] However, a search for attributes or causes obfuscates the social complexity of clinical work by creating an illusion of stable risk and safety characteristics in the system of care.[33]

An understanding of the continuously changing dynamics and unforeseeable complexity of clinical work does not emerge from the precise event sequence constructed by the RCA methodology. The search for root causes is an abstract notion and RCA teams devote lengthy discussions to defining the start and end points of an event.[12] The conversation is frustrated because a causal sequence derived from favorite categories establishes a symmetry that is hard to discern in the reality of messy clinical situations.

The experience of participating on an RCA team is like the moments of uncertainty in the operating room or hospital inpatient unit, where thinking needs to adapt to the situation at hand. Experienced clinicians are quick to see the limitations of causal reasoning in RCA, just as they learn that sorting causal sequences into a taxonomy of disease belongs to medical education more than clinical practice.[30] The practical reasoning of an experienced clinician is necessary on an RCA team where received knowledge is questioned, new possibilities must be considered, and experimentation with alternative ways of working explored: "this means that while physicians (and surgeons) may profess a simple, linear idea of cause and effect, they frequently work as if cause were complex and multifaceted."[30]

The challenge for a hospital executive or policy maker reading an RCA report is that there is no readily available process for controlling future events or predicting how clinicians might respond to uncertain situations. The aggregated reporting of RCA outcomes has more to do with the desire for predictability in processes of health care management than clinical practice. Surgical teams regularly work around the operational limitations of rational organizational plans to safely deliver care. Problems in clinical practice emerge out of complex conditions that could not be predicted in advance.[12] Clinical explanations of adverse events focus on situational responses

Table 2
The VA NCPS RCA triage card of questions

Concepts Used to Identify Contributing Factors	Scope of Questions
Human factors: communication	Flow of information Availability of information Organization's culture of sharing information
Human factors: training	Routine and special job training Continuing education Timing of training Interface between people, workspace, and equipment
Human factors: fatigue/scheduling	Resulting from change, scheduling and staffing issues, sleep deprivation, or environmental distractions Management concern and involvement
Environment/equipment	Use and location of equipment Fire protection and disaster drills Codes, specifications, and regulations Suitability of the environment Possibility of recover after an error
Rules/policies/procedures	Existence and accessibility of directives Technical information to assess risk Feedback mechanisms Interventions developed after previous events Incentives for compliance Qualifications match the level of care provided
Barriers	Protection of people and property from adverse events Barrier strength, fault tolerance, function, and interaction/relationship to rules/policies/procedures and environment/equipment

Available at: http://www.patientsafety.gov/CogAids/Triage/index.html#page=page-1. Accessed December 18, 2011.

rather than stable risk management plans. RCA teams often find it hard to fit their explanations into the language of an RCA report because they know that an "exact failure, in precisely that sequence, will be very unlikely to recur."[33] However, the RCA process tends to focus on the fixable properties of local subsystems and the recommendations are intended to correct the specific issues in the particular adverse event.[34] Successful RCAs look beyond the immediate event and develop recommendations that equip clinicians to respond to similar circumstances and adapt to the unexpected in the clinical workplace.

RESPONDING TO THE LIMITATIONS OF RCA

The RCA process has raised awareness of the need to better manage and respond to adverse events in clinical settings. Many significant problems identified by RCA teams in the last decade have resulted in concerted efforts to better equip clinicians to

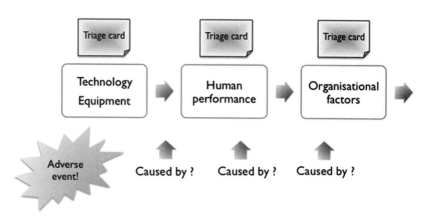

Fig. 1. The constant accident model. The search for causes via triage cards defaults to favorite categories of error. (*Adapted from* Hollnagel E. Thinking about accidents. In: Barriers and accident prevention. Aldershot (United Kingdom): Ashgate; 2004. p. 36–67.)

respond to different categories of safety threats (eg, identification of the deteriorating patient, surgical team briefing, and standardized clinical handover).[35] However, the response to the RCA recommendations is universally uninspiring and many suggestions from RCA teams remain unimplemented.[36,37] RCA is unsuited to capturing the dynamic conditions of the clinical workplace and contrasting perspectives on error and event analysis reinforce this view. It is important to acknowledge that RCA is an incident investigation model with substantial limitations when applied to health care, and to consider alternative tools for the management of serious clinical adverse events. For example, analyzing an event across all levels of an organization by using The London Protocol,[38] or building an understanding of organizational risks through sense making by applying tools that stimulate conversations about processes (eg, failure modes effect analysis) or conversations about system level concerns (eg, probabilistic risk assessment).[39,40]

The different types of accident analysis models (**Table 3**) help to situate the challenges of using RCA to investigate clinical adverse events.[12] The choice of accident model directly influences claims made about the space an event occupies in terms of past experiences, current intentions and relationships, and ongoing constraints on the relations and action in the clinical environment.[41] Integral to the selection of an accident model is appreciating the nature of the event, the complexity of the workplace, the information available for analysis, and the appropriate response given the attributes of the system in place.

A sequential accident model (eg, RCA) is suited to the investigation of events in which there are specific causes and well-defined links and there is a high possibility of eliminating or containing causes.[12] An epidemiologic model looks at an accident in the same way that a clinician describes a disease. The principle behind the inquiry is to discover the factors that combine (ie, performance deviations, environmental conditions, protective barriers, and dormant conditions present in the system before the event).[12] The systemic accident model contrasts the first 2 approaches in that it looks at phenomena that emerge in the normal flow of clinical activity. The systemic model looks for linkages between different interactions that affect performance and constrains the type and level of response to changes in relations in care delivery[12]:

The overriding advantage of systemic models is their emphasis in that accidents analysis must be based on an understanding of the functional characteristics of

Table 3
The assumptions behind different accident models

Accident Model	Objective	Assumption	Response
Sequential model Metaphor: Path	Eliminate or control causes	Cause and effect relationships exist in the adverse event	Search for root causes and contributing factors
Epidemiologic model Metaphor: Net	Identify deviations and implement defenses and barriers	Cause and effect relationships are latent within an organization	Search for the broken components within a broken system
Systemic model Metaphor: Forecast	Monitor and control performance variability	Complex conditions within an organization are emergent and variable	Build foresight to make sense of how system variations function within normal work

Data from Refs. [9,12,23,25,27,33,34]

the system, rather than on assumptions or hypotheses about internal mechanisms as provided by standard representations.[12]

In contrast with the systemic model, which is mostly suited to investigating clinical adverse events, the notion that a sequential accident model like an RCA can be effectively used to find ways to eliminate errors and injuries to patients is limiting.[8] In deference to many investigators in both cognitive psychology and human factors engineering, advocates of RCA in the patient safety movement consider that perfection is the benchmark and competency a central problem in advancing patient safety.[8] This is based on a belief that many doctors have deficiencies that need to be identified and corrected such as deliberate deviation from a known safe practice.[8] Making hospital care safer for patients and ensuring that all clinical disciplines take accountability seriously is laudable, but becoming responsive to the unexpected in the clinical workplace involves the development of competencies and expertise in problem recognition using deliberate practice, and building up a personal catalog of strategies that enable flexibility and adaptability in response to changing circumstances. Learning the basics of error theory, why people make mistakes, and how to prevent them is an academic solution for medical educators, not a practical solution for clinicians in the workplace who have little practical application for error theories.[42]

HAS THE EXCLUSIVE FOCUS ON RCA LED HEALTH CARE ASTRAY?

The introduction of RCA into health care tends to reinforce perceptions of adverse events as reducible to cause and effect, but it has also opened up a space for thinking about the clinical workplace that did not previously exist. Clinicians and managers on RCA teams are engaging in a more conceptual and reflective kind of thinking and talking than they routinely exchange in the operational environment of hospital wards and corridors. RCA teams differ in their interpretation of the incident investigation task but nearly all clinicians express frustration with linear sequencing in the RCA flowcharting exercise. RCA teams develop their view of a particular event by an iterative process, emerging through trial and error over the course of multiple meetings and is often the subject of ongoing debate and discussion beyond the timeframe of the RCA. The features of an adverse event that RCA team members recognize are a concurrence or coincidence[12] of different factors variously combined, but identifiable from similar events in their own clinical and managerial experiences. The past and present experiences of the RCA team members are crucial to the exercise of judgment when interpreting adverse events. The RCA findings are specific to a particular RCA team and group of clinicians with their own mix of habits and routines, conditions of practice, and context-related constraints and disturbances that they must negotiate and adapt to maintain the continuity of care.

CONCLUDING THOUGHTS

The search for causes of patient harm is pervasive in medicine but, when applied to understanding clinician behavior in response to changes in the clinical workplace, it tends to reduce the complexity and produce a reductionist approach of universal explanations independent of the clinical context.[12] The propensity to make general observations is increased by RCA teams because they have limited access to the people involved (usually a single informal interview weeks after the event) and are unable to observe the flow of context-sensitive continuous activity on the day of the event. The RCA team either makes plausible inferences or rejects the exercise outright and does something more meaningful with the RCA meeting space than selecting possible causes. The collective response shifts to trying to make sense of the common experience of clinical work in similar situations.

On many occasions the RCA team decides that there is nothing causal in the event to report but determines to keep meeting anyway: there is a side effect to doing an RCA, which is that it gets people around the table to discuss and explore the deeper issues behind the event.[34] Making sense of what people do in situated contexts is a particular activity,[20] and nothing stimulates it like gathering a small group of clinicians around a complex set of issues. Recognizing the limitations of the RCA process but the associated benefits of structured sense making between clinicians, research by the Institute of Health Improvement (IHI) emphasizes "the importance of studying organizational resilience through structured conversations, in addition to conducting a root cause analysis of adverse events."[21]

We recommend that health care organizations allocate time and resources for surgical teams to participate in structured sense-making conversations with other clinicians. Making sense of complex interactions in the clinical workplace is an inherently concrete and local activity. Engaging frontline staff in this way provides a vital opportunity to scrutinize and improve current practice, influence how recommended actions from improvement activities (such as RCAs) are built into local routines, to identify unnecessary variations in practice, and set precedents for ongoing information gathering, observation, and control of action in the clinical workplace.[39]

There is much that can be learned and applied from the experience of structured clinical conversation during RCAs. The RCA meeting space provides the social context for reflective dialogue that is often hard to find in the midst of busy clinical routines.[43] The confusion and uncertainty around the adverse event provides a focal point for identification. A retrospective glance opens up the opportunity to review past assumptions and make new approximations of safe practice. The small episodes of clinical activity within the adverse event narrative provide cues to the RCA team that come from the edge of routine practice where the unexpected calls for a more flexible response. The situation in the adverse event is not isolated but part of the ongoing flow of clinical activity in the workplace, and the activity of reflection provides the RCA team with improved situational awareness (the individual clinicians in the event are not privy to this rich interaction or outcome). Reflecting on the adverse event helps RCA team members to collectively consider the plausibility of their own practice and routines. The experience of participating on an RCA team affords a small group of clinicians the rare opportunity of working out the best way to adapt to changes in the clinical environment through the enactment of the past adverse event.

A well-facilitated RCA team engages in a rich social form of clinical simulation through the opportunity to enact conditions that other people and other (local) systems have to cope with.[20] Similarly, junior bank tellers are taught to study legal tender notes in detail as opposed to trying to remember all the variations of counterfeit notes presented to the bank in the past. Knowing your clinical workplace and making sense of how your organization fits together and functions is perhaps a more reasonable goal than drafting more rigid rules and policies for preventing errors and controlling risks.

REFERENCES

1. Woodger JH. Causes and causal laws. In: Physics psychology and medicine: a methodological essay. London: Cambridge University Press; 1956. p. 98.
2. Bonacum D, Corrigan J, Gelinas L, et al. 2009 Annual National Patient Safety Foundation Congress: conference proceedings, Lucian Leape Institute town hall plenary: IOM report retrospective and the decade ahead. J Patient Saf 2009;5:131.

3. Bagian JP, Gosbee J, Lee CZ, et al. The Veterans Affairs root cause analysis system in action. Jt Comm J Qual Improv 2002;28:531.

4. Corrigan J, Kohn LT, Donaldson MS, editors. Errors in health care: a leading cause of death and injury. In: To err is human: building a safer health system. Washington, DC: National Academy Press; 2000. p. 26–48.

5. Barach P. The end of the beginning. J Leg Med 2003;24(1):7–27.

6. Streufert S, Satish U, Barach P. Improving medical care: the use of simulation technology. Simul Gaming 2001;32(2):164–74.

7. Berwick D, Rothman M. Pursuing perfection: an interview with Don Berwick and Michael Rothman. Interview by Andrea Kabcenell and Jane Roessner. Jt Comm J Qual Improv 2002;28:268.

8. Leape L. Is hospital patient care becoming safer? a conversation with Lucian Leape. Interview by Peter I. Buerhaus. Health Aff 2007;26(6):687.

9. Dekker S. New frontiers in patient safety. In: Patient safety: a human factors approach. Boca Raton (FL): CRC Press; 2011. p. 213–39.

10. Wu AW, Lipshutz AK, Pronovost PJ. Effectiveness and efficiency of root cause analysis in medicine. JAMA 2008;299:685.

11. Rittel HW, Webber MM. Dilemmas in a general theory of planning. Policy Science 1973;4:155–69.

12. Hollnagel E. Thinking about accidents. In: Barriers and accident prevention. Aldershot (United Kingdom): Ashgate; 2004. p. 36–67.

13. Montgomery K. The misdescription of medicine. In: How doctors think: clinical judgment and the practice of medicine. Oxford (United Kingdom): Oxford University Press; 2006. p. 70–83.

14. Barach P, Berwick DM. Patient safety and the reliability of health care systems. Ann Intern Med 2003;138(12):997–8.

15. Barach P, Johnson JK, Ahmad A, et al. A prospective observational study of human factors, adverse events, and patient outcomes in surgery for pediatric cardiac disease. J Thorac Cardiovasc Surg 2008;136(6):1422–8.

16. Small SD, Barach P. Patient safety and health policy: a history and review. Hematol Oncol Clin North Am 2002;16(6):1463–82.

17. Barach P, Moss F. Delivering safe health care. BMJ 2003;323(7313):585–6.

18. Vincent C, Aylin P, Franklin BD, et al. Is health care getting safer? BMJ 2008;337: a2426.

19. Iedema I, Jorm C. Report on RCA focus groups. In: The evaluation of the Safety Improvement Program, Study 7(b), the Centre for Clinical Governance Research in Health. Sydney (Australia): University of New South Wales; 2005. p. 18–9.

20. Weick KE, Sutcliffe KM, Obstfeld D. Organizing and the process of sensemaking. In: Weick KE, editor. Making sense of the organization, vol. 2. Chichester (United Kingdom): Wiley; 2009. p. 131–51.

21. Conway J, Federico F, Stewart K, et al. Respectful management of serious clinical adverse events, IHI innovation series white paper. Cambridge (MA): Institute for Healthcare Improvement; 2010.

22. Clarke LB. Some functions of planning. In: Mission improbable: using fantasy documents to tame disaster. Chicago: University of Chicago Press; 1999. p. 1–15.

23. Hollnagel E. Accidents and causes. In: Barriers and accident prevention. Aldershot (United Kingdom): Ashgate; 2004. p. 1–35.

24. Cassin B, Barach P. Balancing clinical team perceptions of the workplace: applying 'work domain analysis' to pediatric cardiac care. Prog Pediatr Cardiol, in press.

25. Dekker S. Theorizing drift. In: Drift into failure: from hunting broken components to understanding complex systems. Farnham (United Kingdom): Ashgate; 2011. p. 121.

26. Galvan C, Bacha EA, Mohr J, et al. A human factors approach to understanding patient safety during pediatric cardiac surgery. Prog Pediatr Cardiol 2005;20(1): 13–20.

27. Dekker S. The search for the broken component. In: Drift into failure: from hunting broken components to understanding complex systems. Farnham (United Kingdom): Ashgate; 2011. p. 76–8.

28. Bascetta CA, United States. General Accounting Office. VA patient safety initiatives promising but continued progress required culture change: statement of Cynthia A. Bascetta, Associate Director, Veterans' Affairs and Military Health Care Issues, Health, Education, and Human Services Division, before the Subcommittee on Oversight and Investigations, Committee on Veterans' Affairs, House of Representatives, in testimony; GAO/T-HEHS-00-167. Washington, DC: US General Accounting Office; 2000.

29. Montgomery K. Clinical judgment and the interpretation of the case. In: How doctors think: clinical judgment and the practice of medicine. Oxford (United Kingdom): Oxford University Press; 2006. p. 42–53.

30. Montgomery K. The idea of cause in medical practice. In: How doctors think: clinical judgment and the practice of medicine. Oxford (United Kingdom): Oxford University Press; 2006. p. 57–69.

31. Flin R, O'Connor P, Crichton M. Decision making. In: Safety at the sharp end: a guide to non-technical skills. Farnham (England): Ashgate; 2008. p. 45.

32. Bagian JP, Lee C, Gosbee J, et al. Developing and deploying a patient safety program in a large health care delivery system: you can't fix what you don't know about. Jt Comm J Qual Improv 2001;27:522.

33. Dekker S. Safety culture and organizational risk. In: Patient safety: a human factors approach. Boca Raton (FL): CRC Press; 2011. p. 99–110.

34. Dekker S. The legacy of Newton and Descartes. In: Drift into failure: from hunting broken components to understanding complex systems. Farnham (United Kingdom): Ashgate; 2011. p. 66.

35. Taitz J, Genn K, Brooks V, et al. System-wide learning from root cause analysis: a report from the New South Wales Root Cause Analysis Review Committee. Qual Saf Health Care 2010;19:1–5.

36. Percarpio KB, Watts BV, Weeks WB. The effectiveness of root cause analysis: what does the literature tell us? Jt Comm J Qual Patient Saf 2008;34:391.

37. Morrissey J. Patient safety proves elusive. Five years after publication of the IOM's 'To Err is Human,' there's plenty of activity on patient safety, but progress is another matter. Mod Healthc 2004;34:6.

38. Woloshynowych M, Rogers S, Taylor-Adams S, et al. The investigation and analysis of critical incidents and adverse events in healthcare. Health Technol Assess 2005;9:1.

39. Battles JB, Dixon NM, Borotkanics RJ, et al. Sensemaking of patient safety risks and hazards. Health Serv Res 2006;41:1555.

40. Apostolakis G, Barach P. Lessons learned from nuclear power. In: Hatlie M, Tavill K, editors. Patient safety, international textbook. Faithersburg (MD): Aspen Publications; 2003. p. 205–25.

41. Flach JM, Dekker S, Stappers PJ. Playing twenty questions with nature (the surprise version): reflections on the dynamics of experience. Theor Issues Ergon Sci 2008;9:125.

42. Wears RL. The error of chasing 'errors'. NEFM 2007;58(3):30–31.

43. Waring JJ, Bishop S. 'Water cooler' learning: knowledge sharing at the clinical 'backstage' and its contribution to patient safety. J Health Organ Manag 2010;24:325.

Residency Training Oversight(s) in Surgery: The History and Legacy of the Accreditation Council for Graduate Medical Education Reforms

Russell J. Nauta, MD

KEYWORDS

- Residency training • Surgery • ACGME • Reform

The content and the conduct of a residency in early twentieth century America was largely discipline specific and determined by the sponsoring hospital. By midcentury, the American Board of Medical Specialties (ABMS) and its corresponding residency review committees began to define quality assurance, safety, and educational objectives, which later evolved into the recognizable contemporary guidelines initially administered by the Liaison Committee on Graduate Medical Education, and then by the Accreditation Council for Graduate Medical Education (ACGME).[1]

Aside from unions and collective bargaining, the options for modification of program content and behavior are public centralized regulation, administered by the federal government; public decentralized regulation, administered by a state or region; private decentralized regulation, administered by a practice group or professional society; and private centralized regulation.

The ACGME is a private, centralized regulatory body, whose sudden interest and role in regulating house staff hours was accepted by the surgical community as a 2003 response to the proposed federal (public centralized) legislation proposed earlier that year. Previously, the ACGME had focused on general guidelines common to all graduate medical education programs. Subsequently, exposure of the regulatory shortcomings of public decentralized (state) regulation were highlighted by a high-profile New York case and thrust the ACGME into a more regulatory role.[2]

Department of Surgery, Harvard Medical School, Mount Auburn Hospital, 330 Mount Auburn Street, Cambridge, MA 02138, USA
E-mail address: rnauta@mah.harvard.edu

Surg Clin N Am 92 (2012) 117–123
doi:10.1016/j.suc.2011.12.004
0039-6109/12/$ – see front matter © 2012 Elsevier Inc. All rights reserved.
surgical.theclinics.com

LIBBY ZION AND THE EVALUATION OF ACGME OVERSIGHT OF RESIDENCY TRAINING

The 1984 death of Libby Zion has been extensively analyzed, with general acknowledgment that both the circumstances of her death and her father's prominence as a lawyer and journalist pushed the discourse of the regulation of graduate medical education into the courts and news media. Sidney Zion's teenage daughter died on a teaching service in a New York hospital as a result of drug interactions preventable by a combination of a more detailed admission history and physical, more robust supervision of a postgraduate year 1 (PGY1) resident, and more house staff knowledge of drug interactions. The Bell Commission's duty hour reduction mandates, resulting from investigations of this and similar incidents, were supported by $55 million granted to teaching hospitals from the state of New York, and represented a mandate that was culturally disruptive but funded. However, hospital enthusiasm for enforcing these rules was low. Although oversight of the content of residency training programs by specialty-specific bodies had become commonplace, the overall methodology by which the education was provided differed substantially among specialties and still remained within the purview of the sponsoring teaching hospital. Both specialties and their teaching hospitals clung to their methodology as part of their identity and branding. Traditional stimuli to change, such as challenges to teaching hierarchy, discourse about work hours, or unionization were, in general, foreign to graduate medical education programs, in part because hierarchy, methodology, and culture were discipline specific and intertwined. Moreover, unlike welders, pilots, or truck drivers, residents served in their roles for too short a period of time for true leaders to emerge or for a workers' movement to gain traction.[3]

Thus, the emergence of the ACGME as a private centralized regulatory body is in part based on characteristics of the workforce served, the failure of private decentralized regulatory bodies to unite around common standards, the failure of public decentralized regulation (at least in New York), and the residency programs' fear of public centralized regulation by federal legislation.

TEETH IN THE ACGME REGULATIONS: THE CURRENT SYSTEM

Unlike the New York State mandates of the 1980s, the ACGME mandates regarding work hours are unfunded and imposed without direct financial support from government. The currently high compliance rates with ACGME regulations are rooted in indirect, but potent, stimuli to compliance: funding of residency positions by Medicare and the specialty boards' requirement that candidates for certification be products of an ACGME-accredited program. Acceptance of the changes is driven by the threat of loss of Medicare revenues to support graduate medical education programs and certification ineligibility for the products of noncompliant programs.[2,4]

ALTERNATIVES TO THE CURRENT SYSTEM

The ACGME-induced changes affect the specialty training programs in discipline-specific ways, and many, including surgery, have called for further modification or at least further study.[5,6] An impractical suggestion in a law journal suggests that the general oversight by one private centralized body such as the ACGME is acceptable, but suggests the establishment of regional branches by that body. Such balkanization of oversight, it is argued, theoretically allows creative variations in regulation implementation to occur; best practices would emerge through competition.[2]

This approach is flawed. Applicants to such programs would not only have to consider the intrinsic characteristics of the program but also those of the overseeing body in their choice of residency; for this reason, this approach is impractical. An alternative suggestion has been for specialty-specific societies, such as the American College of Surgeons, to oversee graduate medical education for their respective specialties.[7] This approach requires that the body providing oversight be acceptable to both Medicare and the specialty boards, so that residents would be funded while training and board eligible on completion. Some have opposed this approach as being regressive, returning oversight of postgraduate programs in surgery to a parochial mechanism abandoned in the mid–twentieth century as the Liaison Committee on Medical Education (LCME) and ACGME standards were developed.[8]

EDUCATIONAL RESEARCH: 2 WAVES OF ACGME REGULATIONS

The first round of educational reforms enacted by the ACGME in 2003 stimulated programs to study various methods of compliance and to accumulate data comparing the prereform state of education with the postreform state. Many limited observations were made: increased deaths on orthopedics services before the reform compared with after[6]; more traffic accidents for residents going home after work than for rested residents driving the same distance[9,10]; and motor dysfunction or distraction similar to that imposed by alcohol intoxication[11] or a full urinary bladder (**Box 1**).[12] Some of these limited observations have not been subject to scrutiny as to whether they represent cause and effect, and others are without controls. Still others are methodologically limited by study design or self-reporting of subjective symptoms such as fatigue (**Box 2**).

In response to suggestions made by the Institute of Medicine to further modify work hours, the American College of Surgeons in 2009 suggested that the Institute of Medicine sponsor studies of the relationships between education, fatigue, and safety. Such a study was advocated before further reforms because to study long shifts after the implementation of work-hour restrictions risked disaccreditation.

However, such a study was not done, and further reforms, in particular reforms limiting the number of duty hours worked by an intern to 16, encouraging naps, and further prescribing time off, were required by the ACGME beginning July 2011.

UNANSWERED QUESTIONS AND UNINTENDED CONSEQUENCES

The question of whether the hour modifications adversely or positively affect education or safety remains unanswered, and perhaps unanswerable. However, it should

---

Box 1
Limited observation on the ACGME reforms

- Odds of surgical patient death before and after work-hour restriction: 1.12[6] (meta-analysis of 13 studies)
- Duty hour changes adversely affect student teaching[13] (internal medicine clerkship directors survey)
- Forty-four percent of residents after a call sometimes fall asleep when stopped at a red light[14]
- Residents are slower to intubate after sleep deprivation[15]
- Fewer cases logged per month on q2 night call schedule[16]
- No changes in perioperative complications after a call[15]
- Covered residents on a night float system do not sleep more[17]

Box 2
Studies with self-reporting incorporated into study design

- Residents less happy and less clear thinking after a long night shift[18]
- Affective state declines after 32 hours[19]
- Decreasing work hours increased sleep in the intensive care unit setting[20]
- Medical interns make more errors on shifts longer than 24 hours[21]

---

be possible to answer some questions within the hours constraints imposed by the reforms. Three unintended consequences have been ripe for such study: handoffs of care, the interface of work hours and education, and the potential effect of work hours on patient safety.

SAFETY CULTURE AND HANDOFFS

It has been postulated that any advantage conferred by the presence of a rested resident is negated by the increased frequency of handoffs required when shifts are shortened.

Modern safety culture, as promulgated by the Joint Commission for the Accreditation of Hospitals, has held that hospitals should develop a standardized process for the efficient transfer of information. Nursing and emergency medicine practitioners, for whom shift work is more established, have made early efforts to define the content of a good handoff.[22]

Just as probing a shift length's impact on quality tests the intuitive hypothesis that fatigued residents perform less well than their rested peers, handoff research has sought to verify the inference manifested in the parlor game Telephone, that the more the story is told, the more its specifics are likely to be distorted.[23]

Such testing, focusing on the method of handoff (in person vs video based vs screen based) and the development of computerized patient summary lists, has been the focus of such research. At Johns Hopkins, where the Halstedian ownership model of residency was developed, surgical chief residents have developed 10 essential tools for effective sign-outs.[24] Among these are the designation of adequate time to sign out each patient, the opportunity to question during the sign out, prioritizing a patient such that the sick patients are identified, and precise identification of the supervising senior resident for the upcoming shifts. Standardization of the details of sign out, identification of outstanding tests, laboratories, admissions, and follow-ups complete the list. Computerized tools such as that developed at the University of Washington,[25] which facilitate and reinforce the in-person sign-outs, have been judged to be superior to telephone, video-based, or screen-based alternatives.[26,27]

WORK HOURS AND EDUCATION

Several initiatives developed in New England surgical residencies have attempted to examine the impact of work hours reduction on education. They join the many studies that chronicle the subjective impressions of residents and attending personnel regarding the impact of hours reduction on educational, didactic, and operative experience of the surgical trainee. However, in a large, New England–based study of the objective data provided by American Board of Surgery In-Training Examination scores before and after duty reform, minimal impact was seen after implementation of the duty hours restrictions.[28] These results were similar to those described in an early trial of the 2011 duty hour restrictions on a neurology service, which also showed that both objective and subjective educational experiences were adversely affected by the reforms.[5] More such alternatives to the self-reporting of fatigue and its impact on patient safety are required, with close definition of the subgroups studied. For example, one study conducted on interventions performed before hours reduction has been criticized because the presumed rested residents in all likelihood had an accumulated sleep debt occasioned by hours of wakefulness and did not represent a truly rested control population.[29]

Parshuram[30] has described the difficulties in finding an ideal shift duration, citing individual variability and disagreements as to the impact of fatigue and continuity on patient safety. He has proposed a theoretic framework describing the relationship between increasing shift duration and patient safety. He notes that, if the effects of fatigue and continuity are appropriately counterbalanced, there is no optimal shift duration, whereas an optimal shift duration may be identified if the combined effects result in a U-shaped line. He also notes that currently available data do not support the U-shaped hypothesis (**Fig. 1**).

For every study on a simulator suggesting performance reduction with fatigue, one can be produced showing no difference. Some investigators have documented the broad differences in tolerance of sleep deprivation, going so far as to suggest that certain disciplines may attract or develop individuals with sleep preferences matched to the specialty. A study that required patient error to occur before modifying shift hours would be unethical; however, it is not clear that, on surgical services, fatigue inevitably produces patient harm. Some have attributed this to the high level of supervision inherent on most surgical teaching services; a more cynical view is that even the impaired driver makes it home most of the time.

An increasingly accepted scientific approach is to tie objective neurophysiologic measures to wakefulness to individualize an approach and potentially to define appropriate shifts physiologically. Kahol and colleagues[31] recently studied the performance of simulation tasks over a 4-week period in resident subjects also monitored by electroencephalography. This approach allows for assessment not only of proficiency but of the effects of workload distraction, wakefulness, and attention on task

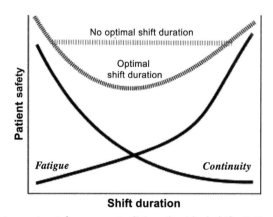

Fig. 1. Parshuram's construct for conceptualizing the ideal shift. Fatigue and continuity reciprocally affect patient shift. If counterbalanced, there is no ideal shift length. If combined effects produce a U-shaped line, for which no evidence exists according to Parshuram, an optimum shift length may be identified. (*From* Parshuram C. The impact of fatigue on patient safety. Pediatr Clin North Am 2006;53:1135–53; with permission.)

performance. Extrapolating from this experience may provide a more data-based approach to the otherwise emotional argument associated with determination of the optimal shift.

SUMMARY

Despite a quarter century of discourse since a sentinel event in New York City raised the question of appropriate oversight for graduate medical education, many questions remain unanswered. Even with the ACGME rules in place, some opportunity remains to examine handoff methodology, the relationship of duty hours to education, and the impact of fatigue on resident performance. Neurophysiologic adjuncts applied concomitantly to evaluation of didactic performance offer some promise for data-driven definition of the optimal shift.

Concurrently, the merits of specialty-specific oversight of graduate medical education, including but not limited to surgical succession from ACGME oversight, remain under active consideration by organizations such as the American College of Surgeons, the Residency Review Committee in Surgery, the American Board of Surgery, and the LCME.[32]

REFERENCES

1. National Center for Health Workforce Information and Analysis. Graduate medical education and public policy: a primer. Washington, DC: US Department of Health & Human Services, US Government Printing Office; 2000.
2. Ciolli A. The medical resident working hours debate: a proposal for private decentralized regulation of graduate medical education. Yale J Health Policy Law Ethics 2007;7(1):175–228.
3. Killelea BK, Chao L, Scarpinato V, et al. The 80-hour workweek. Surg Clin North Am 2004;84(6):1557–72.
4. American College of Surgeons Task Force. Position of the American College of Surgeons on restrictions on resident work hours. Bull Am Coll Surg 2009;94(1): 11–8.
5. Schuh LA, Khan MA, Harle H, et al. Pilot trial of IOM duty hour recommendations in neurology residency programs: unintended consequences. Neurology 2011; 77:883–7.
6. Baldwin K, Namdari S, Donegan D, et al. Early effects of resident work-hour restrictions on patient safety: a systematic review and plea for improved studies. J Bone Joint Surg Am 2011;93(2):E5, 1–9.
7. Nauta RJ. The surgical residency and Accreditation Council for Graduate Medical Education reform: steep learning or sleep learning? Am J Surg 2011; 201:715–8.
8. Flynn TC. Invited comment on: the surgical residency and ACGME reform: steep learning or sleep learning? Am J Surg 2011;202:372–3.
9. Barger LK, Cade BE, Ayas NT, et al. Extended work shifts and the risk of motor vehicle crashes among interns. Harvard Work Hours, Health and Safety Group. N Engl J Med 2005;352(2):125–34.
10. Richardson GS, Miner JD, Czeisler CA. Impaired driving performance in shift-workers: the role of the circadian system in a multifactorial model. Alcohol Drugs Driving 1989-1990;5–6(4–1):265–73.
11. Dawson D, Reid K. Fatigue, alcohol and performance impairment. Nature 1997; 388:235.

12. Lewis MS, Snyder PJ, Pietrzak RH, et al. The effect of acute increase in urge to void on cognitive function in healthy adults. Neurourol Urodyn 2011;30(1):183.
13. Kogan JR, Pinto-Powell R, Brown LA, et al. The impact of resident duty hour reform on the internal medicine core clerkship: results from the clerkship directors in internal medicine survey. Acad Med 2006;81:1338–44.
14. Marcus CL, Loughlin GM. Effect of sleep deprivation on driving safety in house-staff. Sleep 1996;19:763–6.
15. Haynes DF, Schwedler M, Dyslin DC, et al. Are postoperative complications related to resident sleep deprivation? South Med J 1995;88:283–9.
16. Sawyer RG, Tribble CG, Newberg DS, et al. Intern call schedules and their relationship to sleep, operating room participation, stress, and satisfaction. Surgery 1999;126:227–42.
17. Fletcher KE, Underwood W, Davis S, et al. Effects of work hour reduction on residents' lives. JAMA 2005;294(9):1088–100.
18. Leung L, Becker CE. Sleep deprivation and house staff performance: update 1984-1991. J Occup Med 1992;34:1153–60.
19. Bertram DA. Characteristics of shifts and second-year resident performance in an emergency department. NY State J Med 1988;88:10–4.
20. Lockley SW, Cronin JW, Evans EE, et al. Effect of reducing interns' weekly work hours on sleep and attentional failures. N Engl J Med 2004;351(18):1829–37.
21. Landrigan CP, Rothschild JM, Cronin JW, et al. Effect of reducing interns' work hours on serious medical errors in intensive care units. N Engl J Med 2004; 351:1838–48.
22. Varkey P, Karlapudi S, Rose S, et al. A patient safety curriculum for graduate medical education: results from a needs assessment of educators and patient safety experts. Am J Med Qual 2009;24(3):214–21.
23. Zendejas B, Shahzad M, Huebner M, et al. Handing over patient care: is it just the old broken telephone game? J Surg Educ 2011;68(6):465–71.
24. Kemp CD, Bath JM, Berger J, et al. The top 10 list for a safe and effective sign-out. Arch Surg 2008;143(10):1008–10.
25. Van Eaton E, Horvath K, Lober W, et al. A randomized, controlled trial evaluating the impact of a computerized rounding and sign-out system on continuity of care and resident work hours. J Am Coll Surg 2005;200:538–45.
26. Nagpal K, Abboudi M, Fischler L, et al. Evaluation of postoperative handover using a tool to assess information transfer and teamwork. Ann Surg 2011; 253(4):831–6.
27. Bump GM, Jovin F, Destefano L, et al. Resident sign-out and patient hand-offs: opportunities for improvement. Teach Learn Med 2011;23(2):105–11.
28. Sneider EB, Larkin AC, Shah SA. Has the 80-hour workweek improved surgical resident education in New England? J Surg Educ 2009;66(3):140–5.
29. Veasey S, Rosen R, Barzansky B, et al. Sleep loss fatigue in resident training. JAMA 2002;288:1116–24.
30. Parshuram C. The impact of fatigue on patient safety. Pediatr Clin N Am 2006;53: 1135–53.
31. Kahol K, Smith M, Brandenberger J. Impact of fatigue on neurophysiologic measures of surgical residents. J Am Coll Surg 2011;213(1):29–36.
32. Borman KR, Biester TW, Jones AT. Sleep, supervision, education, and service: views of junior and senior residents. J Surg Educ 2011;68(6):495–501.

Teaching the Slowing-down Moments of Operative Judgment

Laurent St-Martin, BSc[a,b], Priyanka Patel, BSc[a,b],
Jacob Gallinger, BA[a],
Carol-anne Moulton, MBBS, MEd, PhD, FRACS[a,c,*]

KEYWORDS

- Control • Expertise • Judgment • Operating room teaching
- Surgical education

With recent changes to educational surgical curricula imposed by increasing standards for patient safety, limited trainee work hours, and increasing budgetary constraints, surgical educators have had to find ways of becoming more efficient and effective teachers. Although the surgical community has found alternative and additional ways of teaching the technical components of surgery, there have been concerns about the adequacy of teaching the more elusive constructs such as judgment as a competency-based training program is adopted. Judgment is poorly understood and lies within the indistinct boundaries of decision making, clinical reasoning, clinical acumen, intuition, and problem solving; although considered essential, the definition of judgment and how it is taught remains poorly understood. The previous training model with training similar to an apprenticeship infused the principles of judgment through long periods of observation and exposure. Efforts are needed to more clearly define judgment and how it might be taught to optimize the current teaching environment.

This work was supported by the Physician Services, Inc.
The authors have nothing to disclose.
[a] The Wilson Centre, University Health Network and University of Toronto, 200 Elizabeth Street, 1ES-565, Toronto, Ontario M5G 2C4, Canada
[b] Institute of Medical Science, University of Toronto, 1 King's College Circle, Room 2374, Toronto, Ontario M5S 1A8, Canada
[c] Department of Surgery, University of Toronto, 100 College Street, Room 311, Toronto, Ontario M5G 1L5, Canada
* Corresponding author. The Wilson Centre for Research in Medical Education, University Health Network and University of Toronto, 200 Elizabeth Street, 1ES-565, Toronto, Ontario M5G 2C4, Canada.
E-mail address: carol-anne.moulton@uhn.on.ca

Surg Clin N Am 92 (2012) 125–135
doi:10.1016/j.suc.2011.12.001
0039-6109/12/$ – see front matter © 2012 Elsevier Inc. All rights reserved.

Recognizing that expert surgeons display good judgment, one of the authors of this article embarked on a PhD to explore a phenomenon identified by surgeons as the hallmark of expertise: the ability to slow down when you should. One of the intentions of this work was to make explicit the implicit construct of judgment.[1] Through the development of a framework to classify the phenomenon of slowing down it becomes possible to understand what is done in surgery that ensures safety. This framework can provide a means for critical reflection and discussion not only about judgment but also about the causes of surgeon error. Furthermore, this framework, as well as an understanding of the control dynamic between surgeon and trainee, provides ways of considering how the teaching of judgment may be facilitated or hindered in the operating room.

THEORETIC FRAMEWORK

First, a brief introduction to the 3 important theoretic perspectives for understanding how surgeons think in practice: attention and effort, situation awareness, and automaticity. These concepts come together in a meaningful way to help understand surgeon behavior and cognition in the development of expertise.

Attention and Effort

In the cognitive psychology literature, there is general agreement that attention capacity is limited (**Fig. 1**).[2] Although attention can be allocated with relative freedom within that capacity, performance suffers once a threshold is reached. The ability to multitask (eg, drive a car, listen to music, and talk on a cell phone) becomes challenged when further stimuli are presented that demand attention (eg, a car turns in front of us). At that stage, attention needs to be reallocated appropriately to the stimuli judged to be most important, or the performance of the primary task suffers.[2]

The operating room is an information-rich environment: the surgical field, monitors, colleagues, and ongoing conversations all vie for attention. As such, the surgeon must selectively attend to certain stimuli. In a critical intraoperative moment, it may be

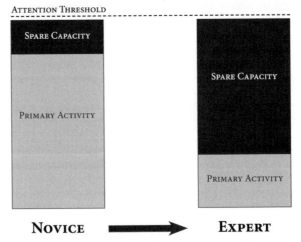

Fig. 1. Availability of attention capacity as a function of experience. Experts develop the ability to perform routine tasks effortlessly, freeing cognitive resources that can be reinvested in other tasks (eg, perceptual monitoring).

necessary to allocate additional attention capacity to the procedure by the sudden removal of a distraction (eg, requesting that the music be turned down). Cognitive capacity that is not presently in use (spare capacity) can be devoted to the perceptual monitoring of one's environment.[2] It therefore follows that, during the critical moments of surgery when spare capacity is limited, the surgeon's ability to detect relevant situational cues is challenged.

Situation Awareness

Situation awareness is defined as the "perception of the elements in the environment within a volume of time and space, the comprehension of their meaning, and the projection of their status in the near future."[3] Put simply, situation awareness is a state of continued understanding in a dynamic environment. Endsley[3] proposed a 3-level hierarchy of situation awareness. Level 1 situation awareness is the perception of relevant environmental features. These features are then interpreted in level 2 to form a global understanding of the current situation. A forecast of the situation is generated for the near future in level 3. The ability to attain and maintain situation awareness in the operative field is crucial to the display of surgical judgment.

The allocation of attention is recognized as involving both bottom-up processes and top-down processes.[4,5] Bottom-up processes are involuntary or spontaneous, first allocating attention to stimuli and establishing meaning and understanding thereafter.[2] For instance, a fast-moving or brightly colored stimulus is likely to be noticed. The sudden appearance of a gush of blood will even be noticed by surgeons who are approaching their cognitive thresholds. Concurrently, top-down processing directs attention to expected perceptual cues.[6] An understanding of the potential dangers in one's environment might therefore cause them to be noticed earlier than if simply relying on bottom-up perceptual processes. For example, a surgeon doing a left colectomy might anticipate and search for the left ureter to prevent incidental injury.

The goals for the task at hand can determine the stimuli that are to be actively sought out.[4] Certain actions are then executed in an effort to align the perceived situation with the desired endpoint. Through the interaction of the various levels of situation awareness, both top-down and bottom-up, a surgeon's understanding of a situation can prompt the revision of planned actions or goals.[3] For example, the general surgeon performing a laparoscopic cholecystectomy might decide to convert to an open procedure in response to a poorly visualized cystic duct.

Schemas facilitate the interpretation of perceived elements.[3] These long-term memory structures store knowledge in a logical and organized manner and are activated by relevant incoming information (pattern recognition).[7,8] They provide a reference point against which comparisons can be made. Schemas emerge with practice,[3] which explains, at least in part, why experience is essential to detect the subtle nuances of a case. Although novices and experts alike might perceive the same situational elements, novices are more likely to incorrectly interpret their significance relative to the task at hand as a result of poorly defined schemas.[3]

Hence, situation awareness is a complex construct that is influenced by many factors, including attention, preconceptions and expectations, goals, and experience. It also plays an important role in surgical judgment, forming the basis for problem naming and framing[9] and decision making, because decisions can be no more sound than the information on which they are made. Many surgeons define judgment as good decision making, and, although this is a part of sound operative judgment, decision making only occurs after the surgeon recognizes a cue, gathers relevant information, and frames the problem in the right context. As an example, a surgeon who clips the bile duct during a gall bladder operation has lost situation awareness; the surgeon did not knowingly decide to clip the bile duct, but rather failed to appreciate the structure as the bile duct.

Automaticity

From the surgeon suturing an incision while talking about his next case to the family physician making the diagnosis of eczema instantaneously, examples of automaticity are common in daily clinical practice. Automaticity is an essential part of competent performance, allowing for the timely and effective resolution of routine problems. In their book *Mind Over Machine*, Dreyfus and Dreyfus[10] argue that this automatic, intuitive approach to practice is the hallmark of expertise. According to their theory, the novice has no intuition or automaticity and simply applies learned rules to situational facts and features. In contrast, experts are largely intuitive. They rarely deliberate, but simply do what normally works. The expert does not assess components of the situation independently, but instead recognizes a holistic pattern, relates it to past experiences, and unconsciously selects and enacts a response.

The benefits of automaticity are clear. The natural performance of a task liberates valuable cognitive resources that can be reallocated to perceptual monitoring (spare capacity; see **Fig. 1**) or any other task (eg, having a conversation with a colleague).[11] However, nobody can perform in a routine mode all the time, and although Dreyfus and Dreyfus[10] allude to unstructured problems, their model of expertise based on automaticity does little to explain how the expert negotiates between the routine and nonroutine aspects of practice.

EXPERTISE IN SURGERY: SLOWING DOWN WHEN YOU SHOULD

Perhaps expert surgical judgment lies neither solely in automaticity nor in reflection, but in an appropriate interplay between these two approaches when necessary. Although the role of automaticity in expertise is obvious, a more deliberate and analytical approach is needed during more critical or uncertain moments to accurately identify and interpret the implications of the problem. In operative practice, the ability to transition from the routine to the effortful through identification of the relevant cues (slowing down when you should[1]) sets apart the expert from the experienced nonexpert,[12] or the adaptive expert from the routine expert (**Fig. 2**).[13]

Manifestations of the Slowing-down Phenomenon in the Operating Room

In previous work, the slowing-down transition was studied in the surgical setting using a qualitative constructivist grounded theory approach. The methodology of these studies has been published elsewhere[14–16] and included interviews with 28 surgeons from varied specialties and observations of 5 hepatopancreatobiliary (HPB) surgeons in the operating room. Four distinct manifestations of the slowing-down phenomenon were identified[15]: stopping, removing distractions, focusing more intently, and fine tuning (from most extreme to most subtle).

In its most extreme form, slowing down is manifested as stopping; the surgeon briefly stops operating in an effort to acquire information needed to move the procedure forward. These stopping moments often reflect some uncertainty on the part of the surgeon, who then seeks out further information (eg, waiting for a second opinion, reviewing the imaging). Some stopping moments are associated with the need to refocus either the individual surgeon or the operative team to an anticipated slowing-down moment. For example, a surgeon might stop the procedure in anticipation of a critical moment to confirm that all members of the surgical team have the correct plan and the necessary equipment to proceed with the next step.

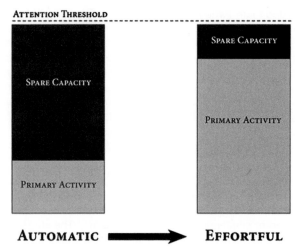

Fig. 2. Reallocation of attention associated with transitioning from the routine to the effortful. The difficult moments of surgery require additional attention, which must be withdrawn from other activities. Spare (unengaged) capacity can be diminished in these moments, increasing the likelihood of missing important perceptual cues.

A less pronounced manifestation is removing distractions: surgeons remove stimuli that they perceive as less important and distracting, and reinvest cognitive resources in the procedure. The distractions are usually in the form of extraneous conversations or music in the background. These distractions were not distracting a few moments before, but suddenly become distracting as the surgeon reallocates attention to the demands that require top priority. Other experienced members of the operative team (eg, a nurse, a fellow) might recognize the surgeons' critical slowing-down moments, removing distracting stimuli on their behalf. Medical students often fail to appreciate these moments, talking through them or otherwise behaving in a seemingly inappropriate manner, simply because they have not yet learned the importance of these transitions and fail to understand the cues that prompt them.

In focusing more intently, the surgeon withdraws from conversations or teaching activities to focus on the surgical field with no attempt to control the noise level or distractions. Surgeons often have telling signs (eg, whistling, tapping a foot) that are noticed by others and that signify that they are in this mode. Less experienced observers may not notice these signs and may try to engage the surgeon in conversations that might not be appreciated.

Fine tuning refers to minor transitions from the routine to the effortful that occur throughout the procedure. Although they occur with high frequency, these moments are so subtle that other members of the operative team might fail to notice them as the surgeon remains engaged in other activities (eg, talking, teaching) with little or no disruption. These transitions are often technically based (eg, readjusting angles or changing procedural techniques) and were suggested to exist during the more routine, or automatic, parts of a procedure for the purpose of staying on track and out of trouble.

Based on the observations in the operating room, the researchers suggested that a varying amount of attention was invested into monitoring activities (using spare capacity) during these more routine or automatic parts of the procedure. Surgeons seemed to be able to deliberately choose what they would do with this spare capacity of attention afforded them through the process of automaticity. They could engage in other conversations or thoughts, or monitor the situation, looking out for relevant or pertinent cues that might alert them that things are not right. The researchers called this a spectrum from inattentive automaticity (with the inherent risk of drifting) to attentive automaticity and suggested that it is a potential source of error during surgery.[15,17]

Regardless of the manifestation, slowing down occurs in an attempt to maintain control over the procedure. In addition, a surgeon does not necessarily progress from fine tuning to stopping in a linear manner. Rather, the extent of slowing down is a reflection of the difficulty or importance of the moment and, by association, of the amount of cognitive resource required to navigate it effectively.

Categorization of the Types of Slowing-down Moments

As surgeons discussed their experiences with slowing down in the operating room, it became apparent that these moments can be divided into 2 broad categories as either proactively planned or situationally responsive (**Fig. 3**).[14] The surgeon either decides before surgery to slow down at a particularly critical moment, or slows down in response to an unexpected critical moment in surgery.

Proactively planned slowing-down moments are determined before entering the operating room. The surgeon reviews the case before surgery and works out an approach to the procedure. The surgeon might be heavily experienced with the case, but plans to slow down every time a particular critical moment is reached. Acknowledging these segments in advance, the surgeon deliberately transitions to an effortful mode of operating when they arise. In this sense, proactively planned moments promote top-down perceptual processing, directing attention to relevant features to help ensure that the procedure goes smoothly.

Proactively planned moments are further divided into 2 categories: procedural-specific moments or patient-specific moments.[14] Procedural-specific moments reflect critical points encountered any time a particular procedure is performed. For example, a surgeon may transition from the routine to the effortful every time the

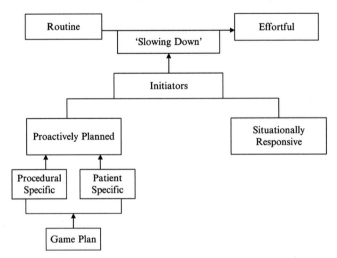

Fig. 3. Conceptual framework for the slowing-down phenomenon. (*From* Moulton CA, Regehr G, Lingard L, et al. 'Slowing down when you should': initiators and influences of the transition from the routine to the effortful. J Gastrointest Surg 2010;14(6):1019–26; with permission.)

superior pedicle is ligated in a thyroid operation. Patient-specific moments are characterized by variations, such as tumor position, abnormal anatomy, or previous surgery, within each patient.

Preoperative planning does not account for surprises in the operating room. Confronted with an unexpected problem (eg, inappropriate planning, unusual anatomy), appropriate slowing down by the surgeon relies on good situation awareness. Consequently, it is said to be situationally responsive. This transition is understood to be a bottom-up cognitive process because the raw input of perceptual data prompts surgeons to realize that they suddenly need to be more attentive.

SLOWING DOWN AND THE SURGEON EDUCATOR

The studies on slowing down presented earlier were conducted in an academic environment; a surgeon's role in a procedure was usually that of supervisor rather than primary operator. These circumstances provided some interesting observations of the manner in which surgeons retain control in the often critical slowing-down moments through the hands of a trainee. Surgeons have competing priorities, ensuring patient safety, but also providing a rich educational experience. It became interesting to consider how this dual responsibility of education and patient safety was reconciled during the slowing-down moments; in particular, it was interesting to see how this negotiation of control around these judgment-rich slowing-down moments might affect the teaching of operative judgment.[16]

The difficulties of maintaining control in a teaching environment are heightened during slowing-down moments. Because these situations require increased effort and attention, and are often masked by some degree of uncertainty, surgeons sense a need to regain control during these moments. The issue of control is understood in terms of direct control and overall control. To distinguish between these potentially confusing levels of control, the term direct control is used to imply levels of manual control, and the term overall control to imply a sense of global control. The amount of direct control retained by the surgeon in charge can vary significantly and is discussed later. In contrast, overall control reflects the surgeons' sense of being in control, whether they are actively or passively participating in the operation.

From an educational standpoint, a willingness on the surgeon's behalf to relinquish direct control to a trainee is necessary. Thus, the surgeon must transfer a certain level of responsibility to the trainee while still preserving a sense of overall control. This giving and taking of direct control is dynamic and managed by the surgeon to balance educational priorities with patient safety priorities. There are other issues in the real-world environment (eg, time restraints), but these can be ignored for the purposes of describing this control dynamic.

Establishing Control

Before surgery, surgeons establish an idea of the level of direct control that will be given to a trainee during a procedure. The decision is based on a global assessment of the trainee's skills, ability to follow directions, and so forth. The trainee's understanding of the case is another important consideration. Staff surgeons are more at ease when they are confident that their trainee is well prepared and has established a plan that emulates their own, anticipating similar potentially critical intraoperative moments. Hence, this general assessment forms the basis for the distribution of direct control between the surgeon and trainee and epitomizes the process of establishing control.

Maintaining Control

The distribution of direct control is constantly negotiated during surgery while surgeon and trainee are scrubbed. Based on the definition of slowing-down moments, both planned and unplanned, as those requiring more attention, the amount of direct control given to the trainee varies throughout the procedure to maintain the surgeon's sense of overall control.

Surgeons have described various strategies used to manage the trainee's direct control of the procedure. For instance, a surgeon may regain control by readjusting the operative view to provide the trainee and surgeon with a different perspective. At a more extreme level, the trainee has the illusion of control; the trainee holds the instruments, but the surgeon has full control of all decision making and technical maneuvering through manipulation of exposure and the art of first assisting. Although this may contribute to a trainee's self-efficacy, it may also instill a false sense of competency when trainees erroneously believe that they had control of the case. As trainees get more senior, they probably start to understand the difference between cases in which they did and did not have direct control. This difference becomes a source of frustration and limited growth if not addressed on an educational level.

TEACHING IMPLICATIONS

The slowing-down taxonomy and framework represent a step forward in the understanding of judgment in the context of surgery. The language enables surgeons to purposefully engage with a phenomenon that previously went unnoticed or was, at the least, difficult to describe. Through an awareness of the concepts of cognitive load and automaticity, surgeons can begin to intentionally monitor their environment to ensure that they slow down when they should. Furthermore, this framework for understanding the slowing-down moments in surgery can be used to help explicitly teach surgical judgment in the operating room.

Teaching the Proactively Planned Slowing-down Moments

All surgeons readily recognize the importance of preoperative planning as a mechanism for promoting sound operative judgment. Planning helps identify both the procedural-specific and patient-specific slowing-down moments, as defined earlier, which ensures that intraoperative surprises are minimized and attention is directed appropriately on the critical moments, facilitating safe and mindful surgery.

However, there is discordance between the recognized importance of planning in surgery and the inclusion of this skill in the surgical curriculum: residents or fellows assisting in a procedure often get no more than a brief look at the patient's chart or computed tomography scan before entering the operating room. Trainees are generally given little opportunity to plan for a case as if it were their own, or "commit" before surgery to a plan that is based on what they perceive to be the relevant information. Demanding a commitment from a trainee in many different teaching contexts has been described as an effective strategy.[18,19] Getting a commitment for the planned slowing-down moments begins to teach the trainees the importance of preoperative planning as well as providing a framework for thinking about it. This plan needs to include their procedural-specific slowing-down moments (ie, every time I do this procedure I will slow down at X, Y, and Z) as well as their patient-specific slowing-down moments (ie, for this particular patient with this particular disorder/anatomy/history, I need to be careful at A, B, and C). Suggesting that they use mental rehearsal and/or visual imagery[20] to make clear their approach to these slowing-down moments has the added advantage of highlighting knowledge or skill gaps and deficiencies that will focus the learner and trainer to these particular moments in surgery. This approach is often ignored in a rushed training environment in which students, trainees, and fellows arrive at the operating room unprepared for the nuances of the operative procedure.

In the context of this slowing-down framework, it can be seen how surgical judgment might be more explicitly taught. As trainees become more senior, their plans should begin to match those of the senior surgeons. Where the plans differ could be informative, becoming the focus of teaching and learning for those particular cases. This focus sets up expectations and clearer objectives, and enables surgeons to teach judgment more explicitly. This approach requires investment from both learner and teacher but, once these expectations are established, it is not overly time consuming and provides a means for optimizing every surgical case.

Teaching the Situationally Responsive Slowing-down Moments

Unplanned or situationally responsive slowing-down moments are valuable teaching opportunities: the recognition of important visual or tactile cues that trigger these transitions, the development of situation awareness in the midst of uncertainty, and the thought processes that occur during these moments all represent vital aspects of surgical judgment. However, these moments are, by definition, not always opportune times for teaching if cognitive demands on the surgeon are high. In these instances, the teaching moment can be delayed until the situation is controlled, but should not be lost completely.

To ensure that the need to slow down is recognized and acted on, surgical training must emphasize the importance of situation awareness of the operative field. Recognition of the important cues develops with experience, but can also be encouraged and stimulated with adequate operative teaching. For trainees, hands-on experience represents a valuable opportunity to develop their own situation awareness and is a prerequisite for understanding the cues that should initiate the slowing-down transition. However, as discussed, hands-on experience varies significantly in its ability to provide the trainee with the control and space that is necessary to develop this situation awareness. Providing trainees with space to develop their own understanding of what is important requires them to have some degree of direct control. This is not feasible when there is concern for patient safety or other more pressing issues, but teachers should be cognizant of how much direct control they are retaining and how much they are giving away. Pressing trainees to commit to what they think is occurring in the operative field provides a picture of how much situation awareness they have and encourages them to be active in the process of continual attainment and maintenance of situation awareness.

The slowing-down framework therefore provides further insight into the competing priorities of the surgeon educator, making apparent the role of critical intraoperative moments in the negotiation of direct control. Understanding the strategies by which a trainee's control of an operation can be managed may enable surgeons to make the transfer of direct control more explicit and rewarding. Simultaneously, an awareness of slowing down as it relates to the control dynamic might encourage the trainee to commit more fully to each case, planning with care and showing an appreciation for potentially important moments. In sum, both surgeon and trainee must understand how operations are controlled from the other's perspective if trainees are to experience the independence needed to develop their situation awareness in the operating room.

SUMMARY

Traditionally, medical education has relied on the assumption that, given enough time, the student will develop the skills and abilities expected of an independent practitioner. However, the surgical community has recently been shifting toward a more structured, competency-based program. The philosophy underlying this new educational paradigm is sensible: by tailoring pedagogy to the achievement of explicit goals and objectives, the educational process should become more effective and efficient. Although motor skill acquisition has been at the forefront of these efforts and advances, concern remains for how this initiative will handle the more elusive competencies, such as surgical judgment. Through the development of this framework and further research to identify ways to effectively teach these slowing-down moments in practice, those concerns can be addressed.

Providing a framework to surgeons that will help them consider more explicitly the vital aspects of surgical judgment may help surgeons and trainees to view judgment not as an obscure and elusive construct, but rather as an object of knowledge that can be modified, molded, and taught in a more explicit and structured way.

REFERENCES

1. Moulton CA, Regehr G, Mylopoulos M, et al. Slowing down when you should: a new model of expert judgment. Acad Med 2007;82:S109–16.
2. Kahneman D. Attention and effort. Englewood Cliffs (NJ): Prentice Hall; 1973. p. 246.
3. Endsley M. Toward a theory of situation awareness in dynamic systems. Hum Factors 1995;37:32–64.
4. Casson RW. Schemata in cognitive anthropology. Annu Rev Anthropol 1983;12: 429–62.
5. Cave KR, Wolfe JM. Modeling the role of parallel processing in visual search. Cognit Psychol 1990;22:225–71.
6. Connor CE, Egeth HE, Yantis S. Visual attention: bottom-up versus top-down. Curr Biol 2004;14:R850–2.
7. Rumelhart DE, Ortony A. The representation of knowledge in memory. In: Anderson RC, Spiro RJ, Montague WE, editors. Schooling and the acquisition of knowledge. Hillsdale (NJ): Erlbaum; 1977. p. 99–135.
8. Custers EJ, Regehr G, Norman GR. Mental representations of medical diagnostic knowledge: a review. Acad Med 1996;71:S55–61.
9. Schön DA. The reflective practitioner: how professionals think in action. New York: Basic Books; 1983. p. 374.
10. Dreyfus HL, Dreyfus SE, Athanasiou T. Mind over machine: the power of human intuition and expertise in the era of the computer. Oxford (United Kingdom): Blackwell; 1986. p. 231.
11. Logan GD. Automaticity, resources, and memory: theoretical controversies and practical implications. Hum Factors 1988;30:583–98.
12. Bereiter C, Scardamalia M. Surpassing ourselves: an inquiry into the nature and implications of expertise. Chicago: Open Court; 1993. p. 279.
13. Mylopoulos M, Regehr G. Cognitive metaphors of expertise and knowledge: prospects and limitations for medical education. Med Educ 2007;41:1159–65.
14. Moulton CA, Regehr G, Lingard L, et al. 'Slowing down when you should': initiators and influences of the transition from the routine to the effortful. J Gastrointest Surg 2010;14:1019–26.

15. Moulton CA, Regehr G, Lingard L, et al. Slowing down to stay out of trouble in the operating room: remaining attentive in automaticity. Acad Med 2010;85:1571–7.
16. Moulton CA, Regehr G, Lingard L, et al. Operating from the other side of the table: control dynamics and the surgeon educator. J Am Coll Surg 2010;210: 79–86.
17. Moulton CA, Epstein RM. Self-monitoring in surgical practice: slowing down when you should. In: Fry H, Kneebone R, editors. Surgical education: theorising an emerging domain. New York: Springer; 2011. p. 169–82.
18. Furney SL, Orsini AN, Orsetti KE, et al. Teaching the one-minute preceptor: a randomized controlled trial. J Gen Intern Med 2001;16:620–4.
19. Neher JO, Stevens NG. The one-minute preceptor: shaping the teaching conversation. Fam Med 2003;35:391–3.
20. Arora S, Aggarwal R, Sirimanna P, et al. Mental practice enhances surgical technical skills: a randomized controlled study. Ann Surg 2011;253:265–70.

The Role of Unconscious Bias in Surgical Safety and Outcomes

Heena P. Santry, MD, MS[a],*, Sherry M. Wren, MD[b,c]

KEYWORDS

- Unconscious bias • Health disparities • Stereotype
- Cognitive processes • Surgical safety

Racial, ethnic, and gender disparities in health outcomes are a major challenge for the US health care system, as highlighted in the landmark Institute of Medicine report, *Unequal Treatment: Confronting Racial and Ethnic Disparities in Health Care* and the Agency for Healthcare Research and Quality's *National Healthcare Disparities Report*.[1,2] Epidemiologic data have demonstrated such disparities for several chronic and acute medical and surgical conditions.[3–31] Although there is evidence that socioeconomic status, access to insurance, overall hospital/physician quality, hospital/surgeon procedure volume, patient/family attitudes, and social networks may explain some of these disparities,[15,32–51] there is no doubt that unequal outcomes are multifactorial in origin and human factors may play a role. One of the most difficult factors to consider is the possible role physicians themselves may play in contributing to these disparities. Most physicians believe that they are socially conscious people who chose a profession where they help people and would never allow prejudices to effect their patient care. In direct contradiction to this self-belief, the Institute of Medicine report identified provider bias and stereotyping as key determinants of "unequal treatment."[1] Health disparities researcher John Ayanian stated, "with a long legacy of racism, segregation, and discrimination in the US society and health care system, overt or

This work was undertaken while Dr Santry was supported by the University of Massachusetts Center for Clinical and Translational Science Clinical Scholar Award funded by grant nos. UL1RR0319821 and KL2RR031981-01 from the National Institutes of Health.
The authors have nothing to disclose.
[a] Department of Surgery, University of Massachusetts Medical School, 55 Lake Avenue North, Worcester, MA 01655, USA
[b] Stanford University School of Medicine, Stanford, CA, USA
[c] Department of Surgery, Palo Alto Veterans Hospital, Stanford University Medical School, G112 PAVAHCS, 3801 Miranda Avenue, Palo Alto, CA 94304, USA
* Corresponding author.
E-mail addresses: Heena.Santry@umassmemorial.org; Heena@santry.org

doi:10.1016/j.suc.2011.11.006
surgical.theclinics.com

subconscious bias among physicians and other health care professionals remains a persistent concern as a potential contributor to racial disparities in care."[52] Disparities have been documented in many areas of surgery, including neurosurgical, orthopedic, cardiothoracic, and vascular, and in general surgical, gynecologic, colorectal, and oncologic outcomes.[4,8,11–13,15,16,19–21,24,25,28,30,31,52–63] Most physicians believe that these disparities have more to do with the systems of care than their own decisions on when and how to provide that care.

According to cognitive psychology research by van Ryn that investigates physician decision making may help explain how well-intentioned physicians can "inadvertently and unintentionally create systematic inequities in health care."[64] Unconscious bias occurs when an individual's subconscious prejudicial beliefs or unrecognized stereotypes about individual attributes, such as ethnicity, gender, socioeconomic status, age, and sexual orientation, result in an automatic and unconscious reaction and/or behavior. Unconscious bias can be measured by the implicit association test (IAT), first described in 1998.[65] The IAT examines automatic associations in memory that are evoked by rapid reactions in response to certain presented features, such as race, gender, age, or sexual orientation.[66] Since originally introduced, the IAT has demonstrated unconscious bias in a multitude of settings.[67] Unconscious bias in the context of health care delivery may result in variable processes of care experienced by patients with similar conditions, resulting in possible disparate outcomes.[68] Surgical outcomes—where the key decision is often whether or not to perform a procedure and the success, failure, or complications from the procedure are the key outcome measures—are perhaps most vulnerable to the effects of unconscious bias.

This article explores the role of unconscious bias as a normative error in surgical performance. Normative error is defined as a situation in which a person fails to carry out his/her moral obligation.[69] Surgeons are obliged to treat patients equally while adhering to the ethical principles of autonomy, beneficence, nonmaleficence, and justice. If unequal treatment occurs as a result of overt or implicit bias, then a normative error has occurred. Understanding and addressing unconscious bias is thus paramount to improving the culture of surgical safety. Theories of social cognition that are at the root of unconscious bias are explored, evidence of unconscious bias in clinical decision making discussed, and recommendations provided to reduce the effects of unconscious bias on surgical outcomes.

WHAT IS UNCONSCIOUS BIAS IN MEDICINE?

Schulman and colleagues' landmark article in 1999[70] put the issue of unconscious bias in clinical decision making at the forefront of American medicine. The article concluded that race and gender influenced physicians' management of chest pain and referral for catheterization. Clinical decision making is a complex process that takes multiple data inputs and should result in similar outcomes if patients' biomedical factors are similar. According to Eisenberg, although physicians "tend to deny the effect of non-biomedical variables" on the care they provide,[71] the clinical steps of physician assessment and initial recommendations are prone to influence by nonbiomedical variables.[71] Einbinder's research has shown that, because clinical recommendations rely on "physician assessment of both tangible and intangible patient characteristics, it is consequently the stage in the referral process at which race-based perceptions and biases about a patient are most likely to enter."[72]

Unconscious bias occurs as part of normal cognitive processing where people's implicit associations can influence their responses to certain tasks, scenarios, medical encounters, and so forth.[68] Thus, physicians are not aware that they are applying stereotypes and prejudices to their decision making. A framework developed by van Ryn[64] outlines 4 possible ways (3 unconscious and 1 conscious) in which providers contribute to racial and ethnic disparities in medical care. This framework could easily be extended to a conceptual model for gender disparities. First, although physicians are expected to make objective decisions based on biomedical data, physicians are no different from all humans who rely on adaptive cognitive processing for decision making. Thus, physicians harbor beliefs about patients that result in the unconscious and automatic projection of stereotype when they make clinical decisions. Second, physicians cognitively classify people and interpret their behaviors through that cognitive lens. Thus, physicians weigh the relative importance of the same reported symptoms and examination findings differently depending on patient history or appearance. Third is the concept of overt moral rationing, wherein physicians consciously make decisions based on their perception of patient qualities, such as likelihood of compliance, social support, and so forth. The fourth possibility arises from physician interpersonal behaviors, which can occur both consciously and unconsciously. Thus, how much eye contact physicians make with a patient, the distance they maintain during the examination, or how forthcoming they are with medical information during discussion may in turn influence patient decisions, compliance, and satisfaction.[64] The majority of researchers exploring health outcome disparities have concluded overt prejudice is rarely a cause of health disparities; rather, unconscious bias is at play.[26,38,64,70,72–75]

EVIDENCE OF UNCONSCIOUS BIAS IN NATURALISTIC STUDIES

It is difficult to deduce the impact of physician decision making on health disparities from so-called naturalistic studies that provide evidence based on observation of real patients, administrative data, or chart review.[76] These data necessarily include measured and unmeasured patient and process variables that may produce disparate outcomes even when no bias is taking effect. Furthermore, most of these studies do not include measures of physician cognitive performance. Nevertheless, many of these real-life research settings and analytic approaches shed some light on the potential role of physician decision making in health care outcomes and provide evidence of unconscious bias.

Although single-center studies may lack generalizability, the study setting is one in which the structure and process of health care delivery can be assumed to be relatively equal across patients. Thus, when these studies find evidence of racial, ethnic, or gender disparities, it is likely physician bias is playing a role. Racial and gender biases have been found in treatment of long bone fractures, HIV treatment, and hormonal replacement therapy at single centers.[77–80] In the surgical domain, disparate outcomes have been demonstrated for varied procedures and diseases, such as transplantation for hepatocellular cancer, amputation versus limb salvage for peripheral vascular disease, and coronary artery bypass surgery for myocardial infarction and angina, each showing preferential care patterns for white patients even though care was delivered at the same center.[56,59,60]

Bach's seminal article in 2002[9] found that, across many cancer types, survival differences between blacks and whites dissipated when patients were comparably treated for similar stage cancers; thus, failure of physicians to treat patients equally after a cancer diagnosis may play a role in racial disparities in long-term cancer outcomes.[9,56,59,60] The Surveillance, Epidemiology and End Results (SEER) program of the National Cancer Institute offers unique insight into the potential role of physician decision making in cancer disparities. In addition to typical epidemiologic, cancer-related, and outcomes data, SEER also records both "referral for treatment" and "treatment rendered," through which variability in type of care delivered may be detected. These outcomes can be measured while simultaneously controlling for sociodemographic factors as well as stage at time of diagnosis. Furthermore, the data can be paired with Medicare claims data for patients over age 65, thus eliminating potential insurance-based confounders on outcomes for older patients as well. SEER data have repeatedly shown that in surgically treatable cancers, such as low-grade gliomas and other brain tumors, squamous cell cancer and adenocarcinoma of the esophagus, and non–small cell lung cancers, blacks have lower rates of surgery compared with whites even when disease stage is equivalent.[8,12,16,18,20,62] These disparities in treatment have also been seen in referral for adjuvant therapy and specific type of operation performed. Blacks with rectal cancer were less likely to receive adjuvant chemotherapy or undergo a sphincter-sparing procedure.[15,19] For patients with locoregional pancreatic adenocarcinoma, blacks were less likely than whites to be referred to a medical, radiation, or surgical oncologist; even after referral they were still less likely to be treated with chemotherapy or surgical resection.[81] Gender disparities have been shown in non–small cell lung cancer patients, where women were less likely than men to be treated with chemotherapy even when controlling for rates of oncologic referral.[82] These SEER data may not explicitly reveal the effect of unconscious bias on these cancer disparities; race, gender, and ethnicity play an important role in types of treatment offered or rendered for cancer treatment.

The Department of Veterans Affairs (VA) health care system provides a setting in which the role of physician bias in treatment can be examined.[83] Within the VA, all of a patient's care is covered through the system. Physicians are salaried and have no financial productivity incentives. Furthermore, all patients are English speaking. These factors should theoretically provide an equal access system for all patients independent of sociodemographic variables. Surprisingly, a review study on racial and ethnic disparities within the VA found several treatment disparities attributable to physician bias.[61] Compared with white veterans, black veterans have been found undertreated for pain due to osteoarthritis, less likely to be offered laparoscopic cholecystectomies well after the safety of the minimally invasive approach had been established, less frequently treated with surgical or interventional revascularization both electively for coronary artery disease (CAD) and for acute myocardial infarction, and less often treated with surgical resection for distal esophageal cancers with similar stage and histology.[45,53,54,58,63,84,85] A large study of patients with peripheral vascular disease found that black race and Hispanic ethnicity were independent risk factors for amputation, even more so than a history of rest pain or gangrene.[86] Even a study that specifically focused on patient attitudes and beliefs determined that physician assessments rather than patient preferences determined rates of referral for coronary revascularization.[87] In studies of other large VA cohorts of colorectal cancer and cerebrovascular disease, however, patients did not reveal any racial disparities in processes of care.[88,89] This suggests that unconscious bias may exist among VA providers but is not universal or the sole explaining factor for the observed disparities.

EVIDENCE OF UNCONSCIOUS BIAS IN EXPERIMENTAL STUDIES

The most compelling data that unconscious bias exists, however, is derived from controlled scientific experiments. Several studies have used survey and vignette data to determine whether or not unconscious bias exists in physician decision making. These methodologies force physician respondents to weigh multiple factors simultaneously and arrive at a clinical decision for a hypothetical patient or case scenario. When race, ethnicity, and/or gender are included in these designs, the results can often provide evidence of unconscious bias. There is ample evidence that vignettes correlate with actual physician practice.[90–92]

Schulman and colleagues'[70] mixed media patient scenarios combining patient complaints of chest pain with various sociodemographic characteristics demonstrated that primary care physicians were equally likely to diagnosis CAD and angina across gender and race variables but they were more likely to refer men and white patients to cardiac catheterization than women or black patients.[70] Another study using video-taped hypothetical scenarios in patient encounters for breast cancer found that older black women needed to behave more aggressively to warrant a more complete staging work-up compared with older white women.[93] Several studies looking at prescribing choices have shown race and gender differences.[74,94,95] Surgical referral for renal transplantation has been shown to be influenced in a similar manner. When the scenario looked at compliant patients, white patients were significantly more likely to be referred for transplantation than black patients. Although noncompliant patients of both races were less likely to be referred for transplantation, the negative effect was stronger among black, noncompliant patients who were least likely of all hypothetical patients to be referred.[96] A similar study of adult nephrologists found that women and Asians were less likely to be referred for kidney transplantation.[97] Some balanced vignette research studies, however, have not found race-based differences in physician decision making for surgical selection of bariatric cases; prescribing practices for hypercholesterolemia, hypertension, and diabetes in primary care; or opioid prescribing practices in the emergency room.[98–102] The reality is perhaps best described by the researchers of a vignette study examining high-risk referral patterns in obstetrics, who noted that, when the clinical evidence was strongly positive or negative in support of a decision, inherent biases had no effect. In this study, Richardson and colleagues found that cases were borderline and close to the high referral threshold, however, were the ones that were "disproportionately susceptible to the marginal influences of numerous personal, social, cultural, and financial considerations."[102] The inference is that unconscious bias may be subtle in obvious clinical situations but in gray areas unconscious bias may perpetuate health disparities.

Gender, race, and ethnicity are just a few potential stereotypes that may trigger unconscious bias in medical decisions. Although less often studied, stereotypical views on patients' personal characteristics, such as reliability, honesty, and so forth, may also bias medical decisions. A multimethod study of interventions for CAD in New York State combining patient race and socioeconomic characteristics in hypothetical scenarios, a survey of both physicians and patients in the postangiogram setting, and data abstraction from actual patient encounters showed that physicians, even when faced with patients sharing the same gender, age, income, and education, were more likely to perceive black CAD patients as less intelligent and at greater risk than white CAD patients for noncompliance, substance abuse, and inadequate social support.[75] Applying similarly complicated analyses to the Medical Outcomes Study data, Safran and coworkers[103] determined that even with equivalent complaints and findings, women were 3.6 times more likely to be prescribed some form of activity limitation compared with men due to gender-based assumptions about baseline activity levels.

The first study using the IAT in medical decision making was published in 2007.[104] The investigators' stated rationale for the study was that "given questions about the source of observed disparities in health service use, the IAT might provide insight into the contribution of implicit biases among physicians." Given the abundant data on disparities in cardiovascular resource use and outcomes, they chose to measure physician decisions on whether or not to give thrombolysis for acute myocardial infarction using a previously validated race-preference IAT and 2 new IATs on general cooperativeness and cooperativeness specifically to medical procedures. The measures of explicit bias showed no differences of physician preference between black and white patients and no variation in attribution of cooperativeness to black and white patients. The measures of implicit bias, however, showed marked differences. Blacks were more strongly associated with negative attributes for all 3 measures. Among patients suspected of having an acute myocardial infarction, black patients were proportionally less likely to be offered thrombolytic therapy. These treatment recommendations correlated with the participants degree of unconscious bias with respondents harboring implicit bias against blacks being more likely to recommend thrombolytic therapy to whites and less likely to do so for blacks.[104] The IAT may serve as an important methodologic tool for the study of unconscious bias in medical decision making.

THE EFFECT OF UNCONSCIOUS BIAS ON THE PHYSICIAN-PATIENT ENCOUNTER

Another manifestation of physician bias can be found when physicians use different communication styles and share different content depending on the race, ethnicity, or gender of a patient. One study of VA patients meeting physicians to discuss findings of coronary angiograms found that physicians were less likely to initiate "information giving" to black patients than to white patients.[105] A multi-institution study exploring hematology malignancy consultations found that "quantitative prognostic discussions without hedging are more likely to occur if the patients are nonwhite."[106] The effect of bias perceived through physician communication style was marked in a study of lung cancer patients treated at a large single VA hospital. Although measured empiric trust in providers was equal between whites and blacks before the encounters, there was notable distrust among blacks compared with whites after they had met with their providers.[107] These same researchers found racially discordant physician-patient relationships to result in more passivity among patients and less information sharing by physicians.[108] Further studies examining physicians' verbal style and body language have shown different approaches used with blacks with whom physicians were observed to be more verbally dominant, less patient centered, and more negative in affect compared with white patients even after controlling for patient-provider racial concordance.[46,109] Peek and colleagues[110] explored black patients' responses to the process of shared decision making (SDM) with their physicians regarding diabetes care. The 3 domains of SDM are information sharing, deliberation and physician recommendation, and decision making. They found that physicians toward blacks compared whites were less likely to actively listen to information sharing, to review treatment options, and to share in the decision-making process.[110] Although sociocultural conditioning may influence how one patient's response to physician communication and behavior differs from another's, these data provide evidence that when observed, physicians themselves, whether or not consciously, communicate and/or behave differently depending on patient race.

REDUCING UNCONSCIOUS BIAS AND IMPROVING SURGICAL SAFETY

Unconscious bias is rarely discussed in the context of surgical safety. Unconscious bias has been well established as an influence in behavior but the question then becomes, Can something be done to ameliorate its effect? Several sociologic and health services researchers have proposed techniques to address this. First there must be conscious acknowledgment that we as physicians and surgeons are all subject to unconscious bias that affects our interactions with patients and our clinical decision making. The Web site, https://implicit.harvard.edu/implicit/, offers a computer-based IAT that individuals can take to explore their unconscious stereotypes and preferences.

Burgess and colleagues[68] provide a conceptual model for reducing unconscious bias by presenting physicians with evidence that bias exists and motivating them to compare what they would do and what they should do when faced with a clinical decision. This works as a self-induced internal motivation instead of external pressure to avoid bias. In reality, physicians and surgeons all already pressure ourselves to avoid socially abhorrent thoughts wherein our stereotypes and prejudices might be apparent. Suppressing these thoughts requires a great deal of cognitive effort and is counter to effectively reducing unconscious bias. Physicians should be educated on the processes of stereotype and prejudice in normal cognition just as they are on the possibilities that human error can occur in an operating room no matter how smart or technically talented they are. One practical approach is use of the IAT for medical student, resident, and faculty training. Post-test debriefing serves as a method of informing providers of their unconscious biases; data show that this alone can result in effective self-regulation of prejudice.[104,111] Acknowledging the existence of stereotype and prejudice on the processing of clinical information is the first step in empowering ourselves to overcome them. The educational approach should be one of promoting equal treatment rather than eliminating bias because this is not likely possible within the developed human psyche.[104,112]

Illness and healing do not occur in a vacuum. Patients' health experiences are shaped by their sociocultural context; stereotypical reactions to a patient's social or cultural milieu can thus perpetuate unconscious bias in health care. Cultural competence is considered an expected skill of modern physicians and has been described as a requirement for physicians who wish to deliver high-quality care to all patients.[113] Even though many physicians may be able to provide the definition of this concept— a professional trait that allows physicians to give empathic, patient-centered care to all patients, including those who are culturally diverse compared with themselves—many practicing physicians have not been educated on how to achieve this in a meaningful way.[113,114] Betancourt[115] has suggested that cultural competence training needs to be more than simple education on attitudes, beliefs, and behaviors typically associated with people sharing particular demographic characteristics. Rather, it should train physicians to explore, on a patient-by-patient basis, the effect of social, cultural, and economic forces on a patient's health-related thoughts and actions.[115] Training in delivering culturally competent care has been shown to improve physician preparedness to treat diverse patient populations.[116] Improved cultural competence among physicians is expected to markedly improve health outcomes across diverse populations.[117] Knowledge of sociocultural context enables surgeons to more broadly measure success after surgery and to develop socioculturally sensitive mechanisms for patient education, selection, and informed consent.

Embracing a patient's sociocultural context requires empathy. Empathy is a powerful tool against unconscious bias. Empathy has been described as a multidimensional tool that incorporates perspective taking, compassion, and a sense of what it is like to be in the patient's position.[68,109,118] Unfortunately, surgeons are not at the top of the scale when compared with other specialists on a validated empathy scale, which may be influenced by the rigors of their training and job.[118,119] Depression, anger, and fatigue have been shown to impair medical trainees' ability to share empathy.[120–122] Burgess suggests that physicians should be mindful of their emotional state; active amelioration of negative emotions has been shown to facilitate empathy and improve patient satisfaction.[68] Higher levels of empathy among medical students have been associated with greater clinical competence.[123] It is reasonable to expect the same effect on the practice of surgery when surgeons embrace an empathic approach to the care of their patients.[68]

As discussed previously, physician communication style is deeply rooted in unconscious bias. Thus, overtly addressing communication is another way to reduce the affects of unconscious bias on medical outcomes. Physicians should be mindful of their use of verbal cues and body language in their patient encounters, in particular with racially, ethnically, or gender-discordant patients. Burgess suggests improving physician confidence in these settings through direct contact with race-discordant colleagues, for example.[68] Physicians who are confident in their spoken and physical approach to patients are less likely to invoke anxiety and mistrust and more likely to engender comprehension of the medical details being provided during the encounter. Johnson proposes a communication curriculum for medical students, residents, and practicing physicians focusing on patient-centeredness and affective dimensions of care.[109] One communication model that has been suggested is SDM.[110,124] In SDM, surgeons empower their patients to tell their story (information sharing), fully disclose the risks and benefits of possible treatment plans, elicit patient preferences for treatment (deliberation and physician recommendation), and finally arrive at a joint decision (decision making).[94,110,111] Irrespective of the exact style, it is likely that a collaborative, patient-centered approach will engender trust. When physicians show concern and put patients at ease while thoughtfully explaining biomedical details, they minimize the distrust that is hypothesized to be at the root of many observed health disparities.[125] Systematic efforts at delivering patient-centered care have been shown to improve outcomes in surgical diseases.[126,127]

There is another type of communication in which unconscious bias may influence surgical safety, namely provider-to-provider communication. To the authors' knowledge no study has examined the role that unconscious bias may play in information transfer between diverse members of a health care team. There have been many studies in the business literature that conclude that gender greatly influences perception of leadership and managerial qualities. It could be speculated that this may translate to implicit discounting of information passed from women to men or women to women. Many female surgeons believe that nurses question their orders more than those of their male colleagues—Could this be an example of unconscious bias? Until the studies are done though there are no data to support or refute the role implicit bias may play in surgical team communications but this is an area that must be explored further to improve the culture of surgical safety.

SUMMARY

Improving surgical safety rests on the reduction of various forms of surgical error. In this article, approaches to the reduction of technical and judgment errors have been addressed. This article shows that surgical and clinical decisions are subject to implicit stereotypes and bias. These subconscious and, therefore, unrecognized errors, although challenging to prove and perhaps even more challenging to ameliorate, present a great risk to surgical safety that must be addressed by the surgical profession in the clinical, teaching, and research settings. Acknowledging unconscious bias, encouraging empathy, and understanding patients' sociocultural context promotes just, equitable, and compassionate care to all patients, both individually and in the aggregate, irrespective of their race, ethnicity, gender, or other personal characteristics.

REFERENCES

1. Unequal treatment: confronting racial and ethnic disparities in health care. Washington, DC: Institute of Medicine; 2003.

2. 2007 National Healthcare Disparities Report. Rockville (MD): Agency for Healthcare Research and Quality, US Department of Health and Human Services; 2008.
3. Ayanian JZ. Heart disease in black and white. N Engl J Med 1993;329(9):656–8.
4. Ayanian JZ, Udvarhelyi IS, Gatsonis CA, et al. Racial differences in the use of revascularization procedures after coronary angiography. JAMA 1993;269(20): 2642–6.
5. Gornick ME, Eggers PW, Reilly TW, et al. Effects of race and income on mortality and use of services among Medicare beneficiaries. N Engl J Med 1996;335(11): 791–9.
6. Allison JJ, Kiefe CI, Centor RM, et al. Racial differences in the medical treatment of elderly Medicare patients with acute myocardial infarction. J Gen Intern Med 1996;11(12):736–43.
7. Ayanian JZ, Weissman JS, Chasan-Taber S, et al. Quality of care by race and gender for congestive heart failure and pneumonia. Med Care 1999;37(12): 1260–9.
8. Bach PB, Cramer LD, Warren JL, et al. Racial differences in the treatment of early-stage lung cancer. N Engl J Med 1999;341(16):1198–205.
9. Bach PB, Schrag D, Brawley OW, et al. Survival of blacks and whites after a cancer diagnosis. JAMA 2002;287(16):2106–13.
10. McBean AM, Huang Z, Virnig BA, et al. Racial variation in the control of diabetes among elderly medicare managed care beneficiaries. Diabetes Care 2003; 26(12):3250–6.
11. Barnholtz-Sloan JS, Schwartz AG, Qureshi F, et al. Ovarian cancer: changes in patterns at diagnosis and relative survival over the last three decades. Am J Obstet Gynecol 2003;189(4):1120–7.
12. Barnholtz-Sloan JS, Sloan AE, Schwartz AG. Relative survival rates and patterns of diagnosis analyzed by time period for individuals with primary malignant brain tumor, 1973-1997. J Neurosurg 2003;99(3):458–66.
13. Barnholtz-Sloan JS, Sloan AE, Schwartz AG. Racial differences in survival after diagnosis with primary malignant brain tumor. Cancer 2003;98(3):603–9.
14. Vaccarino V, Rathore SS, Wenger NK, et al. Sex and racial differences in the management of acute myocardial infarction, 1994 through 2002. N Engl J Med 2005;353(7):671–82.
15. Morris AM, Wei Y, Birkmeyer NJO, et al. Racial disparities in late survival after rectal cancer surgery. J Am Coll Surg 2006;203(6):787–94.
16. Claus EB, Black PM. Survival rates and patterns of care for patients diagnosed with supratentorial low-grade gliomas: data from the SEER program, 1973-2001. Cancer 2006;106(6):1358–63.
17. Lucas FL, Stukel TA, Morris AM, et al. Race and surgical mortality in the United States. Ann Surg 2006;243(2):281–6.
18. Iwamoto FM, Reiner AS, Panageas KS, et al. Patterns of care in elderly glioblastoma patients. Ann Neurol 2008;64(6):628–34.
19. Morris AM, Billingsley KG, Baxter NN, et al. Racial disparities in rectal cancer treatment: a population-based analysis. Arch Surg 2004;139(2):151–5 [discussion: 156].
20. Greenstein A, Litle V, Swanson S, et al. Racial Disparities in Esophageal Cancer Treatment and Outcomes. Ann Surg Oncol 2008;15(3):881–8.
21. Skinner J, Weinstein JN, Sporer SM, et al. Racial, ethnic, and geographic disparities in rates of knee arthroplasty among Medicare patients. N Engl J Med 2003; 349(14):1350–9.

22. Canto JG, Allison JJ, Kiefe CI, et al. Relation of race and sex to the use of reperfusion therapy in Medicare beneficiaries with acute myocardial infarction. N Engl J Med 2000;342(15):1094–100.
23. Dresselhaus TR, Peabody JW, Lee M, et al. Measuring compliance with preventive care guidelines: standardized patients, clinical vignettes, and the medical record. J Gen Intern Med 2000;15(11):782–8.
24. Feinglass J, Kaushik S, Handel D, et al. Peripheral bypass surgery and amputation: northern Illinois demographics, 1993 to 1997. Arch Surg 2000;135(1):75–80.
25. Feinglass J, Rucker-Whitaker C, Lindquist L, et al. Racial differences in primary and repeat lower extremity amputation: results from a multihospital study. J Vasc Surg 2005;41(5):823–9.
26. Curry W, Barker F. Racial, ethnic and socioeconomic disparities in the treatment of brain tumors. J Neurooncol 2009;93(1):25–39.
27. Kressin NR, Petersen LA. Racial differences in the use of invasive cardiovascular procedures: review of the literature and prescription for future research. Ann Intern Med 2001;135(5):352–66.
28. Borkhoff C, Hawker G, Wright J. Patient gender affects the referral and recommendation for total joint arthroplasty. Clin Orthop Relat Res 2011;469(7):1829–37.
29. Irgit K, Nelson C. Defining racial and ethnic disparities in THA and TKA. Clin Orthop Relat Res 2011;469(7):1817–23.
30. Guadagnoli E, Ayanian JZ, Gibbons G, et al. The influence of race on the use of surgical procedures for treatment of peripheral vascular disease of the lower extremities. Arch Surg 1995;130(4):381–6.
31. Steel N, Clark A, Lang IA, et al. Racial disparities in receipt of hip and knee joint replacements are not explained by need: the Health and Retirement Study 1998-2004. J Gerontol A Biol Sci Med Sci 2008;63(6):629–34.
32. Ferris TG, Blumenthal D, Woodruff PG, et al. Insurance and quality of care for adults with acute asthma. J Gen Intern Med 2002;17(12):905–13.
33. Gordon HS, Johnson ML, Ashton CM. Process of care in Hispanic, black, and white VA beneficiaries. Med Care 2002;40(9):824–33.
34. Asch SM, Kerr EA, Keesey J, et al. Who is at greatest risk for receiving poor-quality health care? N Engl J Med 2006;354(11):1147–56.
35. Bach PB, Pham HH, Schrag D, et al. Primary care physicians who treat blacks and whites. N Engl J Med 2004;351(6):575–84.
36. Kahn KL, Pearson ML, Harrison ER, et al. Health care for black and poor hospitalized Medicare patients. JAMA 1994;271(15):1169–74.
37. Eggly S, Harper FW, Penner LA, et al. Variation in question asking during cancer clinical interactions: a potential source of disparities in access to information. Patient Educ Couns 2011;82(1):63–8.
38. Ayanian JZ, Cleary PD, Weissman JS, et al. The effect of patients' preferences on racial differences in access to renal transplantation. N Engl J Med 1999; 341(22):1661–9.
39. Byers TE, Wolf HJ, Bauer KR, et al. The impact of socioeconomic status on survival after cancer in the United States: findings from the National Program of Cancer Registries Patterns of Care Study. Cancer 2008;113(3):582–91.
40. Birkmeyer JD, Siewers AE, Finlayson EV, et al. Hospital volume and surgical mortality in the United States. N Engl J Med 2002;346(15):1128–37.
41. Birkmeyer JD, Stukel TA, Siewers AE, et al. Surgeon volume and operative mortality in the United States. N Engl J Med 2003;349(22):2117–27.
42. Birkmeyer NJ, Gu N, Baser O, et al. Socioeconomic status and surgical mortality in the elderly. Med Care 2008;46(9):893–9.

43. Liu JH, Zingmond DS, McGory ML, et al. Disparities in the utilization of high-volume hospitals for complex surgery. JAMA 2006;296(16):1973–80.
44. Rogers RG. Living and dying in the U.S.A.: sociodemographic determinants of death among blacks and whites. Demography 1992;29(2):287–303.
45. Bradley EH, Herrin J, Wang Y, et al. Racial and ethnic differences in time to acute reperfusion therapy for patients hospitalized with myocardial infarction. JAMA 2004;292(13):1563–72.
46. Horner RD, Oddone EZ, Matchar DB. Theories explaining racial differences in the utilization of diagnostic and therapeutic procedures for cerebrovascular disease. Milbank Q 1995;73(3):443–62.
47. Akerley WL 3rd, Moritz TE, Ryan LS, et al. Racial comparison of outcomes of male Department of Veterans Affairs patients with lung and colon cancer. Arch Intern Med 1993;153(14):1681–8.
48. Ibrahim SA, Siminoff LA, Burant CJ, et al. Understanding ethnic differences in the utilization of joint replacement for osteoarthritis: the role of patient-level factors. Med Care 2002;40(Suppl 1):I44–51.
49. Ho V, Wirthlin D, Yun H, et al. Physician supply, treatment, and amputation rates for peripheral arterial disease. J Vasc Surg 2005;42(1):81–7.
50. Schwartz KL, Crossley-May H, Vigneau FD, et al. Race, socioeconomic status and stage at diagnosis for five common malignancies. Cancer Causes Control 2003;14(8):761–6.
51. Margolis ML, Christie JD, Silvestri GA, et al. Racial differences pertaining to a belief about lung cancer surgery: results of a multicenter survey. Ann Intern Med 2003;139(7):558–63.
52. Ayanian J. Determinants of racial and ethnic disparities in surgical care. World J Surg 2008;32(4):509–15.
53. Arozullah AM, Ferreira MR, Bennett RL, et al. Racial variation in the use of laparoscopic cholecystectomy in the Department of Veterans Affairs medical system. J Am Coll Surg 1999;188(6):604–22.
54. Dominitz J, Maynard C, Billingsley K, et al. Race, treatment, and survival of veterans with cancer of the distal esophagus and gastric cardia. Med Care 2002;40(1):I14–26.
55. Greenberg C, Weeks J, Stain S. Disparities in oncologic surgery. World J Surg 2008;32(4):522–8.
56. Harrison LE, Reichman T, Koneru B, et al. Racial discrepancies in the outcome of patients with hepatocellular carcinoma. Arch Surg 2004;139(9):992–6.
57. Mirvis DM, Burns R, Gaschen L, et al. Variation in utilization of cardiac procedures in the Department of Veterans Affairs health care system: effect of race. J Am Coll Cardiol 1994;24(5):1297–304.
58. Petersen LA, Wright SM, Peterson ED, et al. Impact of race on cardiac care and outcomes in veterans with acute myocardial infarction. Med Care 2002;40(Suppl 1):I86–96.
59. Peterson ED, Shaw LK, DeLong ER, et al. Racial variation in the use of coronary-revascularization procedures. Are the differences real? Do they matter? N Engl J Med 1997;336(7):480–6.
60. Rucker-Whitaker C, Feinglass J, Pearce WH. Explaining racial variation in lower extremity amputation: a 5-year retrospective claims data and medical record review at an urban teaching hospital. Arch Surg 2003;138(12):1347–51.
61. Saha S, Freeman M, Toure J, et al. Racial and ethnic disparities in the VA health care system: a systematic review. J Gen Intern Med 2008;23(5):654–71.

62. Steyerberg EW, Earle CC, Neville BA, et al. Racial differences in surgical evaluation, treatment, and outcome of locoregional esophageal cancer: a population-based analysis of elderly patients. J Clin Oncol 2005;23(3):510–7.

63. Whittle J, Conigliaro J, Good CB, et al. Racial differences in the use of invasive cardiovascular procedures in the Department of Veterans Affairs medical system. N Engl J Med 1993;329(9):621–7.

64. van Ryn M. Research on the provider contribution to race/ethnicity disparities in medical care. Med Care 2002;40(Suppl 1):I140–51.

65. Greenwald AG, McGhee DE, Schwartz JL. Measuring individual differences in implicit cognition: the implicit association test. J Pers Soc Psychol 1998;74(6):1464–80.

66. Plessner H, Banse R. Attitude measurement using the Implicit Association Test (IAT). Z Exp Psychol 2001;48(2):82–4.

67. Greenwald AG, Poehlman TA, Uhlmann EL, et al. Understanding and using the Implicit Association Test: III. Meta-analysis of predictive validity. J Pers Soc Psychol 2009;97(1):17–41.

68. Burgess D, van Ryn M, Dovidio J, et al. Reducing racial bias among health care providers: lessons from social-cognitive psychology. J Gen Intern Med 2007;22(6):882–7.

69. Bosk C. Forgive and remember: managing medical failure. Chicago: The University of Chicago Press; 1979.

70. Schulman KA, Berlin JA, Harless W, et al. The effect of race and sex on physicians' recommendations for cardiac catheterization. N Engl J Med 1999;340(8):618–26.

71. Eisenberg JM. Sociologic influences on decision-making by clinicians. Ann Intern Med 1979;90(6):957–64.

72. Einbinder LC, Schulman KA. The effect of race on the referral process for invasive cardiac procedures. Med Care Res Rev 2000;57(Suppl 1):162–80.

73. Fincher C, Williams JE, MacLean V, et al. Racial disparities in coronary heart disease: a sociological view of the medical literature on physician bias. Ethn Dis 2004;14(3):360–71.

74. Bogart LM, Catz SL, Kelly JA, et al. Factors influencing physicians' judgments of adherence and treatment decisions for patients with HIV disease. Med Decis Making 2001;21(1):28–36.

75. van Ryn M, Burke J. The effect of patient race and socio-economic status on physicians' perceptions of patients. Soc Sci Med 2000;50(6):813–28.

76. Elstein AS, Holmes MM, Ravitch MM, et al. Medical decisions in perspective: applied research in cognitive psychology. Perspect Biol Med 1983;26(3):486–501.

77. Todd KH, Deaton C, D'Adamo AP, et al. Ethnicity and analgesic practice. Ann Emerg Med 2000;35(1):11–6.

78. Todd KH, Samaroo N, Hoffman JR. Ethnicity as a risk factor for inadequate emergency department analgesia. JAMA 1993;269(12):1537–9.

79. Moore RD, Stanton D, Gopalan R, et al. Racial differences in the use of drug therapy for HIV disease in an urban community. N Engl J Med 1994;330(11):763–8.

80. Schneider AE, Davis RB, Phillips RS. Discussion of hormone replacement therapy between physicians and their patients. Am J Med Qual 2000;15(4):143–7.

81. Murphy M, Simons J, Ng S, et al. Racial differences in cancer specialist consultation, treatment, and outcomes for locoregional pancreatic adenocarcinoma. Ann Surg Oncol 2009;16(11):2968–77.

82. Earle CC, Neumann PJ, Gelber RD, et al. Impact of referral patterns on the use of chemotherapy for lung cancer. J Clin Oncol 2002;20(7):1786–92.

83. Oddone EZ, Petersen LA, Weinberger M, et al. Contribution of the Veterans Health Administration in understanding racial disparities in access and utilization of health care: a spirit of inquiry. Med Care 2002;40(Suppl 1):I3–13.

84. Dominick KL, Dudley TK, Grambow SC, et al. Racial differences in health care utilization among patients with osteoarthritis. J Rheumatol 2003;30(10):2201–6.

85. Peterson ED, Wright SM, Daley J, et al. Racial variation in cardiac procedure use and survival following acute myocardial infarction in the Department of Veterans Affairs. JAMA 1994;271(15):1175–80.

86. Collins TC, Johnson M, Henderson W, et al. Lower extremity nontraumatic amputation among veterans with peripheral arterial disease: is race an independent factor? Med Care 2002;40(1):I106–16.

87. Kressin NR, Chang BH, Whittle J, et al. Racial differences in cardiac catheterization as a function of patients' beliefs. Am J Public Health 2004;94(12):2091–7.

88. Dominitz JA, Samsa GP, Landsman P, et al. Race, treatment, and survival among colorectal carcinoma patients in an equal-access medical system. Cancer 1998;82(12):2312–20.

89. Oddone EZ, Horner RD, Johnston DC, et al. Carotid endarterectomy and race: do clinical indications and patient preferences account for differences? Stroke 2002;33(12):2936–43.

90. Langley GR, Tritchler DL, Llewellyn-Thomas HA, et al. Use of written cases to study factors associated with regional variations in referral rates. J Clin Epidemiol 1991;44(4–5):391–402.

91. Peabody JW, Luck J, Glassman P, et al. Comparison of vignettes, standardized patients, and chart abstraction: a prospective validation study of 3 methods for measuring quality. JAMA 2000;283(13):1715–22.

92. Alexander C, Becker H. The use of vignettes in survey research. Public Opin Q 1978;33:93–104.

93. Krupat E, Irish JT, Kasten LE, et al. Patient assertiveness and physician decision-making among older breast cancer patients. Soc Sci Med 1999;49(4):449–57.

94. Weisse CS, Sorum PC, Dominguez RE. The influence of gender and race on physicians' pain management decisions. J Pain 2003;4(9):505–10.

95. Weisse CS, Sorum PC, Sanders KN, et al. Do gender and race affect decisions about pain management? J Gen Intern Med 2001;16(4):211–7.

96. Furth SL, Hwang W, Neu AM, et al. Effects of patient compliance, parental education and race on nephrologists' recommendations for kidney transplantation in children. Am J Transplant 2003;3(1):28–34.

97. Thamer M, Hwang W, Fink NE, et al. U.S. nephrologists' attitudes towards renal transplantation: results from a national survey. Transplantation 2001;71(2):281–8.

98. Santry HP, Lauderdale DS, Cagney KA, et al. Predictors of patient selection in bariatric surgery. Ann Surg 2007;245(1):59–67.

99. Rathore S, Ketcham J, Alexander G, et al. Influence of patient race on physician prescribing decisions: a randomized on-line experiment. J Gen Intern Med 2009;24(11):1183–91.

100. Tamayo-Sarver JH, Dawson NV, Hinze SW, et al. The effect of race/ethnicity and desirable social characteristics on physicians' decisions to prescribe opioid analgesics. Acad Emerg Med 2003;10(11):1239–48.

101. Freund KM, Moskowitz MA, Lin TH, et al. Early antidepressant therapy for elderly patients. Am J Med 2003;114(1):15–9.

102. Richardson DK, Gabbe SG, Wind Y. Decision analysis of high-risk patient referral. Obstet Gynecol 1984;63(4):496–501.
103. Safran DG, Rogers WH, Tarlov AR, et al. Gender differences in medical treatment: the case of physician-prescribed activity restrictions. Soc Sci Med 1997;45(5):711–22.
104. Green A, Carney D, Pallin D, et al. Implicit bias among physicians and its prediction of thrombolysis decisions for black and white patients. J Gen Intern Med 2007;22(9):1231–8.
105. Gordon HS, Street RL Jr, Kelly PA, et al. Physician-patient communication following invasive procedures: an analysis of post-angiogram consultations. Soc Sci Med 2005;61(5):1015–25.
106. Alexander SC, Sullivan AM, Back AL, et al. Information giving and receiving in hematological malignancy consultations. Psychooncology 2011. DOI: 10.1002/pon.1891. Available at: http://onlinelibrary.wiley.com/doi/10.1002/pon.1891/abstract;jsessionid=B6C89B9F877D84443BA332139152ABDD.d02t04?systemMessage=Wiley+Online+Library+will+be+disrupted+3+Dec+from+10-12+GMT+for+monthly+maintenance. Accessed November 17, 2011.
107. Gordon HS, Street RL Jr, Sharf BF, et al. Racial differences in trust and lung cancer patients' perceptions of physician communication. J Clin Oncol 2006; 24(6):904–9.
108. Gordon HS, Street RL Jr, Sharf BF, et al. Racial differences in doctors' information-giving and patients' participation. Cancer 2006;107(6):1313–20.
109. Johnson RL, Roter D, Powe NR, et al. Patient race/ethnicity and quality of patient-physician communication during medical visits. Am J Public Health 2004;94(12):2084–90.
110. Peek ME, Odoms-Young A, Quinn MT, et al. Race and shared decision-making: perspectives of African-Americans with diabetes. Soc Sci Med 2010;71(1):1–9.
111. Devine PG, Plant EA, Amodio DM, et al. The regulation of explicit and implicit race bias: the role of motivations to respond without prejudice. J Pers Soc Psychol 2002;82(5):835–48.
112. Burgess DJ, Warren J, Phelan S, et al. Stereotype threat and health disparities: what medical educators and future physicians need to know. J Gen Intern Med 2010;25(Suppl 2):S169–77.
113. Betancourt JR. Cultural competence—marginal or mainstream movement? N Engl J Med 2004;351(10):953–5.
114. Betancourt JR, Green AR, Carrillo JE, et al. Cultural competence and health care disparities: key perspectives and trends. Health Aff (Millwood) 2005; 24(2):499–505.
115. Betancourt JR. Cultural competence and medical education: many names, many perspectives, one goal. Acad Med 2006;81(6):499–501.
116. Lopez L, Vranceanu AM, Cohen AP, et al. Personal characteristics associated with resident physicians' self perceptions of preparedness to deliver cross-cultural care. J Gen Intern Med 2008;23(12):1953–8.
117. Betancourt JR, Green AR. Commentary: linking cultural competence training to improved health outcomes: perspectives from the field. Acad Med 2010;85(4):583–5.
118. Hojat M, Gonnella JS, Nasca TJ, et al. Physician empathy: definition, components, measurement, and relationship to gender and specialty. Am J Psychiatry 2002;159(9):1563–9.
119. Hojat M, Gonnella JS, Nasca TJ, et al. The Jefferson Scale of Physician Empathy: further psychometric data and differences by gender and specialty at item level. Acad Med 2002;77(Suppl 10):S58–60.

120. Bellini LM, Baime M, Shea JA. Variation of mood and empathy during internship. JAMA 2002;287(23):3143–6.

121. Bellini LM, Shea JA. Mood change and empathy decline persist during three years of internal medicine training. Acad Med 2005;80(2):164–7.

122. Hojat M, Mangione S, Nasca TJ, et al. An empirical study of decline in empathy in medical school. Med Educ 2004;38(9):934–41.

123. Hojat M, Gonnella JS, Mangione S, et al. Empathy in medical students as related to academic performance, clinical competence and gender. Med Educ 2002; 36(6):522–7.

124. Peek ME, Tang H, Cargill A, et al. Are there racial differences in patients' shared decision-making preferences and behaviors among patients with diabetes? Med Decis Making 2011;31(3):422–31.

125. Collins TC, Clark JA, Petersen LA, et al. Racial differences in how patients perceive physician communication regarding cardiac testing. Med Care 2002; 40(1):l27–34.

126. Anderson GD, Nelson-Becker C, Hannigan EV, et al. A patient-centered health care delivery system by a university obstetrics and gynecology department. Obstet Gynecol 2005;105(1):205–10.

127. Brown JB, Stewart M, McWilliam CL. Using the patient-centered method to achieve excellence in care for women with breast cancer. Patient Educ Couns 1999;38(2):121–9.

When Bad Things Happen to Good Surgeons: Reactions to Adverse Events

Shelly Luu, BSc[a,b], Shuk On Annie Leung, BASc[a,b], Carol-anne Moulton, MBBS, MEd, PhD, FRACS[a,c,*]

KEYWORDS

- Adverse events • Judgment • Psychological reactions
- Surgeon wellness

VIGNETTE

Tom Sinclair is an active 56-year-old professor of engineering recently diagnosed with colorectal cancer. Eager to find the best surgeon around, Tom asked advice from a friend, a nurse on your surgical ward, who recommended he see you. He came to your office with his wife of 30 years and was relieved that you recommended surgery the week after. He said he would delay a preorganized family holiday he was taking with his wife and 3 children to get this surgery behind him. As he left the office, you thought how difficult this diagnosis must be for him briefly imagining how you might feel if you received the same news. You are not that different in age after all, and the thought of dying at such a young age was a little too difficult to imagine. It was a fairly straightforward operation with no signs that the cancer had spread elsewhere. The tumor was a little lower in the rectum than you expected, but you decided that a covering stoma was not necessary, so you performed the anastomosis and closed. Tom's wife and 3 teenaged children were waiting in the operating room as you walked in to tell them the good news.

This work was supported by the Ministry of Research and Innovation Early Researcher Award and the Royal College of Physicians and Surgeons of Canada Medical Education Research Grant.

[a] The Wilson Centre for Research in Medical Education, University Health Network and University of Toronto, 200 Elizabeth Street, 1ES-565, Toronto, Ontario M5G 2C4, Canada

[b] Faculty of Medicine, University of Toronto, 1 King's College Circle, Room 2109, Toronto, Ontario M5S 1A8, Canada

[c] Department of Surgery, University of Toronto, 100 College Street, Room 311, Toronto, Ontario M5G 1L5, Canada

* Corresponding author. The Wilson Centre for Research in Medical Education, University Health Network and University of Toronto, 200 Elizabeth Street, 1ES-565, Toronto, Ontario M5G 2C4, Canada.

E-mail address: carol-anne.moulton@uhn.on.ca

Surg Clin N Am 92 (2012) 153–161
doi:10.1016/j.suc.2011.12.002
0039-6109/12/$ – see front matter © 2012 Published by Elsevier Inc.

"Thank-you doctor. You are our lifesaver," his daughter said. You saw him every day, and each time he and his family were very grateful to you, singing your praises. You were a little embarrassed but accepted this acknowledgment as a great perk of your job. On the sixth postoperative day, you were called by the resident who had been on the night before to let you know that he thought Mr Sinclair—"your colon" from last week—was leaking. Tom had deteriorated overnight with sudden onset of abdominal pain and fevers, and his blood pressure dropped. He had a low-grade fever the day before, but you thought it was from a little redness at the wound site. You had removed a few staples and thought he should be fine. "How do you know he has leaked?" you asked somewhat agitatedly. A computed tomographic scan was just performed, which showed large amounts of free air and fluid throughout Tom's abdomen and particularly in his pelvis. You hang up the phone.

Adverse events are unfortunately a part of every surgical practice. As surgeons who are intimately linked to these events, they affect each one of us, although the exact nature and impact of these events have not been well articulated or understood. Studies that have attempted to characterize the surgical personality from a psychological perspective have found that surgeons form the most distinct and consistent group among physicians.[1] As a group, surgeons are trained for rapid and confident decision making with little room for error[2] and reside in a culture where disclosure of error and explicit discussion of their own personal causes for error are not always facilitated.[3] Surgical residents experience internal conflict as they are taught about the uncertainty of medicine in parallel with the unacceptability of error[4] and, as opposed to other professions, counseling or debriefing at the individual level after medical errors is not routine.[3] Moreover, surgeons are often reluctant to disclose errors to patients and colleagues for fear of malpractice litigation,[5] shame, or self-disappointment.[6] In-depth interviews conducted with general internists have found that error, whether perceived or real, reduced physicians' self-confidence and induced fear of stigmatization and feelings of guilt.[7] The competitiveness of medical practice, belief in physician control, and the basic principle of "first, do no harm" were noted to explain physicians' responses to medical errors.[3]

During a recent qualitative study as part of a larger program of research exploring surgical judgment, surgeons described considerable physiologic and psychological reactions when things went wrong.[8] Surgeons would say, "I remember all my deaths," or "We all have our own graveyard," with details of these events seemingly burned in their memory.[9] This seemed to be in contradiction to a previous discussion in the literature that suggested surgeons experience fewer symptoms of distress than internists[10] and surgeons are more willing to risk failure.[11] Given how relatively little is known about surgeons' reactions to such events, we embarked on another qualitative study to explore this phenomenon in surgical practice. Terminology in this area is confusing in the current literature, with some terms (eg, error or mistake) having negative connotations associated with fault or, worse, negligence and others (eg, complication or adverse event) implying acts of God.[12,13] It is often difficult to elicit the exact cause of an adverse event and therefore difficult to ever fully appreciate one's exact role in the event. Was this an error or an act of God, a complication that would have happened no matter what in the best of hands because of this invasive intervention? This difficulty sets up a period of rumination of 'was it my fault,' which is described later.

In this article, we present a framework to understand surgeons' reactions to adverse events, which were derived from a more recent study (details and methodology have been presented elsewhere)[9] as well as a review of both the relevant psychology and social psychology literatures that helped guide us in our understanding of these reactions. We situate this framework within the broader picture of mindful practice to gain an appreciation of how the psychological and social dimensions of the surgeon can affect judgment and cognition.

FRAMEWORK FOR UNDERSTANDING INDIVIDUAL SURGEONS' REACTION TO ADVERSE EVENTS

Surgeons who participated in the study were reported to believe that their own reactions to adverse events were unique and relieved to hear that colleagues experienced similar reactions. Interesting differences were described when men attributed their reactions to being outliers (eg, when compared with their colleagues), whereas women attributed their reactions to being women (eg, more emotional, less ego). The investigators suggested that participants were aware that external appearances during these reactions may not be congruous with what was being experienced on the inside. Surgeon's culture promotes strength and certainty, and demonstrations of vulnerability or self-doubt are discouraged. When participants interviewed surgeons who had been described by their peers as cold or seemingly unaffected by these reactions, they found these individuals suffered similar reactions to adverse events. Given the consistency of these reactions, the investigators were able to define 4 phases that occurred among surgeons: *kick, fall, recovery, and long-term impact.*[9]

4 PHASES OF REACTION TO ADVERSE EVENTS
The Kick

The first phase that was described in this study was the *kick*; when surgeons first heard news of the event, they experienced a physiologic stress or anxiety reaction. There were physical manifestations of this phase, such as tachycardia, sweatiness, and agitation, which was reported to last up to several hours. The investigators also described significant feelings of failure that seemed complicated by not only sadness for the patient but also sadness for how it made them feel personally.[9] Surgeons described feeling like they were no longer worthy of being a surgeon, likening it to getting a "D" on a test rather than the expected and usual "A."[9] Several factors were identified that influenced the severity of the reaction: the age of the patient, the nature of the case (emergent vs elective), the relationship they had developed with family and friends, and the severity of the complication.[9] The dissonance surgeons felt between striving to be the ideal perfect surgeon and the current adverse event led to exaggerated emotions and self-blame.[9]

The Fall

After the *kick*, the next phase was described as the *fall*, when surgeons felt a downward spiral of emotions as they tried incessantly to find out details of the case in the hope that they would be somewhat exonerated in the complication. In this phase, surgeons questioned almost every aspect of the case to answer the question, "Was it my fault?"[9] Long periods of rumination to uncover the details of the case were described.[9] Although blame was not a big part of this phase, participants recognized the tendency to blame in an attempt to feel better about the situation.

Although surgeons put forth an ardent effort to find out whether they were responsible for the adverse event, it was often difficult to exactly discern the cause of the adverse event, let alone determine the role they played. Surgeons were more distressed if they felt they had contributed in some way to the adverse event. The uncertainty resulted in extended periods of information searching and an inability to focus on other tasks.[9]

The Recovery

The beginning of the *recovery* phase was marked by a return of feeling normal and undistracted by the thoughts of failure associated with the first 2 phases. Surgeons described being able to continue with their daily work with ruminating thoughts of the event finally controlled. In brief interviews with surgeons after events, the investigators noted that surgeons were calmer and more reflective during the recovery phase. One surgeon was said to describe this as "the pall has lifted." Surgeons realized the need to recover and move on from the event.[9]

Surgeons had different coping strategies to deal with the adverse events in their recovery phase, including discussion with colleagues and family. It seemed that surgeons felt better able to cope with the event once they satisfied themselves that they learned something from the event that will prevent future occurrences. One surgeon described changing the standard of practice after every adverse event, whereas another noted that teaching residents about the adverse event was a way of coping.[9]

The Long-Term Impact

Even though surgeons experienced adverse events similarly in the short-term period, there seemed to be differences in the cumulative effect of these reactions over time. Several surgeons suggested the *long-term impact* was a negative one, recognizing that these reactions were not getting any better or easier to handle with time. Several suggested that these reactions were actually getting worse and became the primary factor for considering early retirement or changing their scope of practice.[9] These surgeons felt that the negative effect of these reactions over many years of their practice was cumulative, perhaps understandably when it is not uncommon to hear surgeons say, "I remember all my deaths by name." An understanding of the severity of these reactions in the acute phase coupled with an understanding of the surgical culture sheds light on this statement.

IMPLICATIONS: PLACING THE FRAMEWORK INTO CONTEXT

The framework for understanding surgeons' reaction to error illustrates the consistency with which surgeons experience adverse events. Translating this knowledge to promote patient safety in surgery requires an examination of the external or social environment that surgeons operate in as well as the internal landscape and cognitive processes inside the surgeon's head.

The surgical culture stresses certitude, decisiveness, and confidence.[14] In the acute phase after an adverse event has occurred, surgeons described the need to manifest these qualities of strength despite experiencing powerful negative emotions—to put on a brave face. Thus there is a tension between needing to appear strong and actually being strong after a complication.

The sociology literature describes social identity as an aspect of an individual's self-concept that is derived from the individual's membership in a group[15]; a surgeon's professional identity, therefore, is derived from belonging to the larger social group formed by health care practitioners.[16] When there is incongruence between personal and professional identity, for example, feeling vulnerable and imperfect after a surgical complication, identity dissonance is created.[17] The pressure to conform to mainstream expectations around behaviors, attitudes, and belief systems is well documented in health care trainees entering training programs as well as individuals who are not part of the mainstream (eg, cultural/religious minorities, women in predominantly male environments).[17–19] In the following sections, guided by various literatures, we examine the framework for surgeons' reaction to error in the context of the surgical culture and its various implications as we strive for safer surgery.

Operating After a Complication

"I honestly think I almost crashed into four parked cars before I got out of the parking garage that day. I was so distraught…" (I-002).[9]

The first 2 stages, the kick and the fall, were described as incapacitating for many surgeons because they found it difficult to concentrate on other activities during this period.[9] Looking at the cognitive psychology literature on human attention, it suggests that a limited cognitive capacity exists for paying attention.[20–22] Humans have a limited space of attentional resources, and, once that threshold is reached, the mind tends to take mental shortcuts and oversimplify at the cost of accuracy. As nicely captured in the aforementioned quotation, the ability to think straight after the recognition of a significant adverse event might be compromised. Although "crashing into four parked cars"[9] in this state is an extreme example, it exposes the potential for how these reactions might interfere with subsequent judgment and decision making, particularly in the operative setting. In any intraoperative moment, there are numerous external and internal stimuli that are in essence competing for the surgeon's attention (see the article by Carol-anne Moulton and colleagues elsewhere in this issue). The ability to think clearly and gather and process information at the moment of crisis can be jeopardized by consuming thoughts and emotions associated with ruminating on a previous complication.

Learning from Adverse Events: Reactions as a Source of Feedback

Learning from surgical errors and complications occur at both macrolevels and microlevels. At the macrolevel, systems-based initiatives such as surgical checklists are a result of recognized patterns of errors.[23,24] At the microlevel, individual surgeons also learn to refine their procedural techniques and decision making from their errors. Furthermore, it has been suggested that emotion-laden reactions to errors that are subjective, variable, and surgeon dependent are also an important source for learning.[25]

Surgeons vividly described emotions, and their physiologic manifestations, during the kick phase. These strong emotions are actually a powerful form of feedback for learning in addition to other formal system-implemented sources of feedback. It has been hypothesized that intuition comes from emotions and sensory input that are packaged with experiences and form part of our memory; when the memory is retrieved, the emotions and sensory experiences are automatically retrieved, often influencing behavior and decision making.[26,27] Neurocognitive research has shown that subcortical areas, especially those involved in emotion and reactions to threat, process information beneath conscious awareness, and the input from these areas directly shapes reasoning.[28] Therefore, the strong emotions evoked by a complication become imprinted in the memory of the surgeon, having the potential to influence decision making in subsequent cases in which this memory is retrieved unconsciously.

Counterfactual thinking is another psychological concept relevant to learning from adverse events. It describes the process of asking oneself questions such as what if or if only, comparing actual outcomes with imagined alternatives.[29] Surgeons commonly engage in counterfactual thinking in response to a complication, particularly in the information-gathering or the fall phase. Counterfactual thinking can be either upward (better than reality) or downward (worse than reality) and also outward focused (outside of my control) or self-focused (within my control).[29] In the context of how surgeons interpret adverse events, counterfactuals that are both downward (it could have been worse) and outward focused (it is out of my control) are effective coping mechanisms but may lead to minimization of the event and blame (eg, other colleagues, systems factors).[29] On the other hand, self-focused upward comparisons are more likely to result in performance-promoting learning (eg, if I had checked the blood work again before operating, this adverse event may have been avoided).[30]

Surgeons might use counterfactual thinking in their reflections on adverse events. The pancreatic surgeon who resects a tumor resulting in positive oncological margins may use the upward counterfactual, "It doesn't matter; a positive margin doesn't always result in rapid local recurrence and death." Alternatively, the surgeon may use the following downward counterfactual after the same error: "It could be worse; the patient may have died from a leaking pancreatic anastomosis." Counterfactual thinking and emotions associated with the event both serve as feedback for critical reflection on personal performance.[31] It has been suggested that for feedback to be effective, it should be specific, directed, and task oriented rather than self-oriented.[31] However, the paradox is that surgeons' sense of self or personal identity is inextricably linked to their professional identity and performance as a surgeon.[32] Poor outcome after surgery, particularly if attributable to surgeon error, can provide negative feedback on surgeon performance in self-assessment. This feedback, which is both inconsistent with and lower than self-perceptions, can elicit negative emotions in the surgeon. There are many psychological and neurocognitive mechanisms in place to counteract negative feedback that surgeons receive.[33] Becoming aware of these mechanisms might improve the potential for learning through critical self-reflection around the event.

Why Error Disclosure is Difficult

An American professor of law, Carol Liebman, asked if it was possible to train physicians to communicate better with their patients, with an end goal of improving and facilitating error disclosure.[34] After 2 years of research, the investigator concluded, "We're putting good people in positions where no one can succeed. Communicating with patients in these situations is just too difficult." She further explained, "It's just too hard for physicians who are facing emotional turmoil themselves" and that "physicians operate in a system in which the culture does not give them much space to process their feelings."[35]

The social pressures associated with the culture of decisiveness and certainty in surgery contributes directly to the difficulties in disclosure. Physicians are often reluctant to disclose errors to patients and superiors because of fear of malpractice litigation,[5] shame and sense of inadequacy, and also high expectations of themselves.[36] The official institutional forum for the discussion of adverse events, Morbidity and Mortality Conferences, has been evaluated with ambivalence by residents who are detracted by the threat of remediation and fear of getting "toasted" by colleagues.[37]

In addition to the social pressures, results from our study also provide insight into why error disclosure is so difficult from the perspective of negative emotions.[9] It has been found that disclosing self-focused counterfactuals can imply (incorrectly) to others that the surgeon was negligent or culpable in the adverse event. Therefore, it is less likely that individuals performing under organizational accountability pressures (such as surgeons under pressure of Morbidity and Mortality Rounds) would use such counterfactuals immediately after an adverse event,[30] especially when they are immediately distressed. This is unfortunate because self-focused upward counterfactuals are the type of counterfactuals that are conducive to learning. Immediate reactions may be the reason why physicians do not learn as much from Morbidity and Mortality Rounds as hoped.[38,39]

FUTURE DIRECTIONS AND SUMMARY

The 4 phases of surgeons' reaction to error characterizes the surgeon as the second victim and might be a causative factor in the rising levels of surgeon depression and burnout.[11] The reaction can be profound and is consistent across surgeons of different genders, experience levels, and specialties.[9] Little research has been done in the way of evaluating support measures for physicians undergoing distress from adverse events.[40] It has been suggested that by modifying the medical curriculum, increasing mentoring, and ultimately changing the culture in which adverse events are understood, it may be possible to lessen the emotional distress that physicians will encounter in the future.[11] By increasing the surgical community's awareness and understanding of the pervasiveness and severity of surgeons' reactions to error, the culture can be made more accommodating and discussions with colleagues can be facilitated. Furthermore, special attention needs to be paid to surgical residents and fellows to prepare them for their future roles as attending surgeons because the new roles with greater responsibility for patients can result in greater distress in the event of error.[39]

One way surgeons may better understand and process their own reaction and its potential impact on subsequent judgment is to develop the habits of what Epstein and others[41] have described as mindful practice, the definition of which is the "conscious and intentional attentiveness to the present situation." Applying the 4 habits of the mind, attentive observation, critical curiosity, beginner's mind, and presence, when surgeons are experiencing these reactions allows surgeons to become more aware of their emotions and performance at the moment.[41–43] As mentioned previously, the strong emotions evoked by a complication become imprinted in the memory of the surgeon, having the potential to influence decision making in subsequent cases as this memory is retrieved, sometimes subconsciously. It has been shown in a study with primary care physicians that mindful practice can be taught,[44] offering benefits of not only reflective abilities at the moment but also personal well-being.[45]

The framework presented in this article can serve as a platform for healthier and more productive discussions about adverse events and errors. It has been suggested, "the language people use both makes possible and constrains the thoughts they can have. More than just a vehicle for ideas, language shapes ideas—and the practices that follow from them."[46,47] With the language provided by this framework, it might be possible to better prepare and train the future generation of surgeons for what to expect when adverse events occur. It is quite possible that once surgeons learn they are not alone in these reactions and have a language to discuss them and a background to understand them, the negative impact of these reactions might be mitigated.

REFERENCES

1. Coombs R, Fawzy F, Daniels M. Surgeons' personalities: the influence of medical school. Med Educ 1993;27(4):337–43.
2. Sexton JB, Thomas EJ, Helmreich RL. Error, stress, and teamwork in medicine and aviation: cross sectional surveys. BMJ 2000;320(7237):745–9.
3. Rowe M. Doctors' responses to medical errors. Crit Rev Oncol Hematol 2004; 52(3):147–63.

4. Leape LL. Error in medicine. JAMA 1994;272(23):1851–7.
5. May T, Aulisio MP. Medical malpractice, mistake prevention, and compensation. Kennedy Inst Ethics J 2001;11(2):135–46.
6. Charles V, Nicola S, Margaret CM. Reasons for not reporting adverse incidents: an empirical study. J Eval Clin Pract 1999;(1):13–21.
7. Christensen JF, Levinson W, Dunn PM. The heart of darkness: the impact of perceived mistakes on physicians. J Gen Intern Med 1992;7(4):424–31.
8. Moulton CA, Regehr G, Lingard L, et al. "Slowing down when you should": initiators of the transition from the routine to the effortful. J Gastrointest Surg 2010; 14(6):1019–26.
9. Luu S, Leung S, Regehr G, et al. Waking up the next morning: surgeons' reactions to adverse events, in press.
10. Vaillant GE, Sobowale NC, McArthur C. Some psychologic vulnerabilities of physicians. N Engl J Med 1972;287(8):372–5.
11. Newman MC. The emotional impact of mistakes on family physicians. Arch Fam Med 1996;5(2):71–5.
12. Chan DK, Gallagher TH, Reznick R, et al. How surgeons disclose medical errors to patients: a study using standardized patients. Surgery 2005;138(5):851–8.
13. Espin S, Levinson W, Regehr G, et al. Error or "act of God"? A study of patients' and operating room team members' perceptions of error definition, reporting, and disclosure. Surgery 2006;139(1):6–14.
14. Good MJ. American medicine, the quest for competence. Berkeley (CA): University of California Press; 1995.
15. Gergen KJ, Davis KE. The social construction of the person. New York: Springer-Verlag; 1985.
16. Dryburgh H. Work hard, play hard: women and professionalization in engineering—adapting to the culture. Gend Soc 1999;13(5):664–82.
17. Monrouxe LV. Identity, identification and medical education: why should we care? Med Educ 2010;44(1):40–9.
18. Beagan BL. "Even if I don't know what I'm doing I can make it look like I know what I'm doing": becoming a doctor in the 1990s. Can Rev Sociol Anthropol 2001;38(3):275–92.
19. Costello CY. Professional identity crisis: race, class, gender, and success at professional schools. Nashville (TN): Vanderbilt University Press; 2005.
20. Kahneman D. Attention and effort. Englewood Cliffs (NJ): Prentice-Hall; 1973.
21. Cowan N, Elliott EM, Scott Saults J, et al. On the capacity of attention: its estimation and its role in working memory and cognitive aptitudes. Cognit Psychol 2005; 51(1):42–100.
22. Moray N. Where is capacity limited? A survey and a model. Acta Psychol (Amst) 1967;27:84–92.
23. Haynes AB, Weiser TG, Berry WR, et al. A surgical safety checklist to reduce morbidity and mortality in a global population. N Engl J Med 2009;360(5):491–9.
24. Reason J. Safety in the operating theatre—part 2: human error and organisational failure. Qual Saf Health Care 2005;14(1):56–60.
25. Sargeant J, Mann K, Sinclair D, et al. Understanding the influence of emotions and reflection upon multi-source feedback acceptance and use. Adv Health Sci Educ Theory Pract 2008;13(3):275–88.
26. Damasio AR. The feeling of what happens: body and emotion in the making of consciousness. New York: Harcourt Brace; 1999.
27. Schmidt HG, Norman GR, Boshuizen HP. A cognitive perspective on medical expertise: theory and implication. Acad Med 1990;65(10):611–21.

28. Porges SW. Love: an emergent property of the mammalian autonomic nervous system. Psychoneuroendocrinology 1998;23(8):837–61.
29. Kahneman D, Miller DT. Norm theory: comparing reality to its alternatives. Psychol Rev 1986;93(2):136–53.
30. Morris M, Moore P. The lessons we (don't) learn: counterfactual thinking and organizational accountability after a close call. Adm Sci Q 2000;45:737–65.
31. DeNisi A, Kluger A. Feedback effectiveness: can 360-degree appraisals be improved? Acad Manage Exec 2000;14(1):129–39.
32. Pratt M, Rockmann K, Kauffmann J. Constructing professional identity: the role of work and identity learning cycles in the customization of identity among medical residents. Acad Manag J 2006;49(2):235–62.
33. Festinger L. A theory of cognitive dissonance. Evanston (IL): Row, Peterson and Company; 1957.
34. Liebman CB, Hyman CS. A mediation skills model to manage disclosure of errors and adverse events to patients. Health Aff (Millwood) 2004;23(4):22–32.
35. Why physicians need help when talking about serious errors. Today's Hospitalist 2004. Available at: http://todayshospitalist.com/index.php?b=articles_read&cnt=368. Accessed July 15, 2011.
36. Vincent C, Moorthy K, Sarker SK, et al. Systems approaches to surgical quality and safety: from concept to measurement. Ann Surg 2004;239(4):475–82.
37. Schwappach DL, Koeck CM. What makes an error unacceptable? A factorial survey on the disclosure of medical errors. Int J Qual Health Care 2004;16(4):317–26.
38. Orlander JD, Fincke BG. Morbidity and mortality conference: a survey of academic internal medicine departments. J Gen Intern Med 2003;18(8):656–8.
39. Wu AW, Folkman S, McPhee SJ, et al. Do house officers learn from their mistakes? Qual Saf Health Care 2003;12(3):221–6 [discussion: 227–8].
40. Schwappach DL, Boluarte TA. The emotional impact of medical error involvement on physicians: a call for leadership and organisational accountability. Swiss Med Wkly 2009;139(1–2):9–15.
41. Epstein RM, Siegel DJ, Silberman J. Self-monitoring in clinical practice: a challenge for medical educators. J Contin Educ Health Prof 2008;28(1):5–13.
42. Borrell-Carrio F, Epstein RM. Preventing errors in clinical practice: a call for self-awareness. Ann Fam Med 2004;2(4):310–6.
43. Epstein RM. Mindful practice. JAMA 1999;282(9):833–9.
44. Krasner MS, Epstein RM, Beckman H, et al. Association of an educational program in mindful communication with burnout, empathy, and attitudes among primary care physicians. JAMA 2009;302(12):1284–93.
45. Siegel DJ. The mindful brain. New York: WW Norton; 2007.
46. Burke K. A rhetoric of motives. Berkeley (CA): University of California Press; 1969.
47. Lingard L, Haber RJ. Teaching and learning communication in medicine: a rhetorical approach. Acad Med 1999;74(5):507–10.

Open Disclosure of Adverse Events: Transparency and Safety in Health Care

Aaliyah Eaves-Leanos, JD, PhD[a], Edward J. Dunn, MD, ScD[b,c],*

KEYWORDS

- Disclosure • Transparency • Patient safety • Ethics
- Professional • Legal

In the Veterans Health Administration (VHA), adverse events are defined as untoward incidents, iatrogenic injuries, or other adverse occurrences resulting in patient harm directly associated with care or services provided within the jurisdiction of a medical center, outpatient clinic, or other medical facility. The phrase disclosure of adverse events refers to the forthright and empathetic discussion of clinically significant facts between providers or administrators and patients or their personal representatives about the occurrence of a harmful adverse event, or an adverse event that could result in harm in the foreseeable future.[1]

Disclosure of adverse events can be counterintuitive to physicians, especially if there was no suspicion of any problem in health care delivery perceived by the patient. Why invite trouble? In the past, the practice of medicine supported by professional medical societies and health care organizations advised physicians to remain silent on these matters or limit discussions to their malpractice defense attorneys and hospital administration when things went wrong. Health care organizations, spurred on by the acrimonious relationship between the legal and medical professions, frequently denied and defended the occurrence of an adverse event.

A consequence of this institutionalized secrecy was patient confusion and fear about what was happening and what the future held for their health and well-being. At a time when a patient and family needed their health care providers the most, they were adversaries. Patients and their families resorted to legal means when left with more questions than answers and a growing suspicion that the physician was not telling the whole story. The American College of Surgeons Closed Claim Study

The authors have nothing to disclose.

[a] Lexington VA Medical Center, Lexington, KY, USA
[b] Lexington VA Medical Center, 1101 Veterans Drive, Lexington, KY 40502-2236, USA
[c] Department of Health Policy & Management, College of Public Health, University of Kentucky, 111 Washington Avenue, Lexington, KY 40536-0003, USA
* Corresponding author. 703 Braeview Road, Louisville, KY 40206.
E-mail addresses: Edward.dunn@va.gov; edwdun@gmail.com

Surg Clin N Am 92 (2012) 163–177
doi:10.1016/j.suc.2011.11.001
0039-6109/12/$ – see front matter Published by Elsevier Inc.

surgical.theclinics.com

showed a significant association between tort claims and the lack of transparency between surgeons and their patients.[2] Reducing the patient and provider adverse event experience to a lawsuit exacerbates the unmet expectations of both parties and, in some cases, furthers harmful consequences from health care.

This article rejects the old paradigm of silence and secrecy following an adverse event and makes the case for open disclosure of adverse events to patients and their families as part of the routine practice of medicine. Adverse event disclosure to patients should be part of the expected course of managing a health system, without exception. We establish the ethical, professional, and legal basis for disclosure and share our perspectives on how to operationalize disclosure in the practice of medicine and in the standard operations of managing a medical center in the VHA.

WHY DISCLOSE ADVERSE EVENTS?

In 1987, the Chief of Staff of the Lexington Veterans Affairs Medical Center (VAMC) and the Staff Attorney for the US Department of Veterans Affairs (VA) Regional Counsel Office in Lexington, Kentucky, discovered that a patient had succumbed from a mistake made in the medical care provided in their facility. They made the decision to disclose what happened to the family, who had no knowledge of this mistake in care, because it was the right thing to do. At that moment, the humanistic risk management program, called the Lexington Model, was born.[a,3]

Steve Kraman and Ginny Hamm, who had the courage and vision to see the wisdom of honesty and transparency as the most effective means of managing adverse events in health care, started the informal practice of disclosure with patients. In Lexington, when an adverse event occurred, there would be an early case review, full disclosure in a face-to-face meeting with the patient and/or family, an authentic apology with acceptance of full responsibility by the organization for what happened, an offer of fair compensation, and sharing of an action plan to prevent a similar occurrence in the future. Over the following 23 years, Lexington continued to have tort claims (Lexington ranked in the top quartile of tort claims among VAMCs), but they also ranked in the bottom quartile for litigation costs.[4]

The humanistic risk management approach envisioned by the Lexington VAMC was not driven by a rationale that open disclosure in health care prevents lawsuits, but rather the desire to facilitate just outcomes for patients and providers. Just outcomes as a moral good in this context emanate from the ethical, professional, and legal duties health care professionals owe to their patients.

THE ETHICAL OBLIGATION FOR DISCLOSURE

In *Principles of Biomedical Ethics*, Beauchamp and Childress[5] outline 4 principles of bioethics that offer a common morality approach to health care ethics by eliminating contentious or marginally relevant metaphysical concepts and distilling the basic common moral framework held by persons with differing belief systems. This approach to health care ethics, also known as principalism, establishes specific duties

---

[a] In 1987, after losing 2 malpractice judgments totaling $1.5 million, senior management of the Lexington VAMC decided to become more proactive with investigating clinical cases with the potential for tort claims and be better prepared for defending against those claims. In the course of investigation, there were several cases in which negligent care had been delivered that was unknown to the patient's next of kin. The Lexington Risk Management team was confronted with an ethical dilemma that they resolved by meeting with the family to inform them what had happened: that negligent care contributed to the death of their loved one. The Lexington Model of humanistic risk management was born.

owed by medical providers and, by negative implication, bestows associated rights on patients. Arguably, the 4 principles of autonomy, nonmaleficence, beneficence, and justice form the foundation for all generally accepted ethical norms in health care and apply to all patients and members of the medical profession.[5]

The duty to respect patients' rights to direct the course of their own moral lives and make medical decisions is encompassed in the principle of autonomy. The duty to provide benefits that are reasonable in relation to the risks of medical treatment and the correlated rights of patients to have their medical providers act for their benefit is the principle of beneficence. The principle of nonmaleficence is described as a patient's right to be free from avoidable harm at the hands of the medical provider and the duty of the provider to avoid causing harm. The duty to be fair in the distribution of benefits and risks is the justice principle, which corresponds with the patient's right to receive a fair and equitable share of benefits and burdens.

Numerous professional societies codify medical providers' ethical requirement to disclose adverse events to patients in accordance with the common morality approach of the 4 principles, including the American College of Physicians' Ethics and Human Rights Committee,[6] the International Council of Nursing,[7] and the American Medical Association (AMA).[8] Of particular note is the influential moral imperative contained in the AMA Code of Medical Ethics. The code states that "It is a fundamental ethical requirement that a physician should at all time deal honestly and openly with patients... Only through full disclosure is a patient able to make informed decisions regarding future medical care... Concern regarding legal liability that might result following truthful disclosure should not affect the physician's honesty with a patient."[8]

The principle of autonomy is contained in the AMA's ethics code when it counsels medical professionals to provide truthful information about patient care in order for patients to make future medical decisions. The principles of beneficence and justice are shown by the requirement to put patients' interests before their own concern for legal liability, thus ensuring that patients do not shoulder the burden of the adverse events alone. The duty of nonmaleficence applies even after the harm caused by the adverse event, because the provider could exacerbate harm by not being honest with the patient about what happened.

Our experience in Lexington VAMC with disclosure of adverse events to patients or their personal representatives is not only consistent with these ethical norms, it is also informed by our organizational ethics, which are derived from our commitment to care for veterans. The VHA as a health care provider has a fiduciary responsibility to its patients, employees, affiliates, and the communities in which it exists. The organizational core values of integrity, commitment, advocacy, respect, and excellence guide our employees and institutional leaders. Honestly discussing the difficult truth that an adverse event has occurred shows respect for the patient and a commitment to improving care.

PROFESSIONAL DUTY

Similar to the VHA's institutional responsibility to its patients by virtue of its position, health care providers have a fiduciary duty to disclose adverse events to their patients. This duty is inherent in the health care profession's contract with society. The health care professional has expert knowledge, training, and technical skills that the public must trust will be applied to enhance their health and well-being. Information asymmetry between the medical profession and the community places the medical provider in the role of the patient's fiduciary. Trust is a critical element to the success of the therapeutic relationship.

The high degree of privilege that society has bestowed on the health profession carries the expectation that the profession will be self-regulating with standards established to benefit patients. The health profession has been permitted the latitude to regulate the practice of medicine by defining education requirements, granting or revoking licenses to practice, and forming medical specialty societies to establish standards of care. The act of professionalism is to uphold the standards that are defined by the profession.

Professional standards include being truthful and trustworthy, treating all patients respectfully and without bias, and avoiding conflicts of interest. Michael Woods,[9] a Colorado General Surgeon, defines professionalism as commitment, caring, and competence. In his words, "acting in a professional manner includes offering an apology when there has been an unexpected outcome... Apology is about the provider showing respect, empathy, and a commitment to patient satisfaction."[9] Clinical and administrative staff members have a professional duty to protect the welfare of patients by preserving and supporting appropriate professional behavior. Therefore, disclosure of adverse events to patients should be a routine part of patient care.

LEGAL AND REGULATORY MANDATE

Any breach of professional standards of care that result in patient harm, including the failure to disclose, qualifies for legal remediation. Patients have a fundamental right to prevent unwanted bodily interference. This concept, called the doctrine of informed consent, grants a qualified legal right to competent patients to direct what happens to their bodies. In turn, health care professionals have a legal right to collect fees for services they provide and a legal obligation to refrain from nonconsensual medical contact with patients. To ensure that the contact between the parties is consensual, medical providers have an affirmative duty to involve patients in a process of shared decision making for all medical treatments and procedures. Providers also have an affirmative duty to inform patients of all relevant facts about their treatment so that they can make decisions that are consistent with patients wishes and values.

In the case of an unexpected outcome, such as an adverse event, the patient has the right to be informed about the event with its implications to current and future health. Without full and open disclosure, patients may be unable to make informed consensual decisions, including whether or not they wish to continue treatment with their providers. Withholding information or misleading patients about relevant medical information violates patients' legal right to bodily integrity and may even breach contractual duties between the parties.

The legal and regulatory duty to disclose any aspect of medical care that affects a patient's health and well-being has been mandated by several states, accreditation bodies, licensing boards, federal regulations, and national policies.[10] The Joint Commission, which is funded to accredit more than 80% of health care organizations, expresses this rule through the following language: "The responsible licensed independent practitioner or his or her designee clearly explains the outcome of any treatment or procedure to the patient and, when appropriate, the family, whenever those outcomes differ significantly from the anticipated outcomes."[11] The VHA, which is the largest integrated health care system in the United States, issued a national directive establishing a specific mandate for full and open clinical, institutional, and large-scale disclosure for adverse events.[1]

DISCLOSURE LINK TO PATIENT SAFETY

Ethical, professional, and legal duties that health care professionals owe to their patients after adverse events often overlap. When the question is framed as a conflict of interest between patients" right to know and the providers' or institutions' desire to limit liability or reputational harm, there is a strong presumption in favor of open and honest disclosure.[12] Another argument for open disclosure of adverse events is the advancement of patient safety goals.

Those who choose to draw a line between patient safety and risk management claim that patient safety is focused on systems improvements and learning and that risk management is focused on individual accountability including tort claim management. However, such linear, one-dimensional thinking is not the reality of a modern health care system. Risk management and patient safety are both focused on the risk to the safety and well-being of patients in health care delivery. The 2 terms are linguistically interchangeable in patient-centered organizations and, in the reality of health system operations, they must be fully integrated for optimal patient care.

Patient safety should not be limited to an engineering problem focused only on systems solutions. When a patient has suffered injury as a result of health care, the injured patient's needs are paramount. The patient safety zealots have often preached the mantra of systems while leaving the injured patient's needs in the background. Carol Levine[13] addressed this problem: "Medical error is more than an engineering problem amenable to technological and systems solutions. Policies put in place to reduce medical error also must address the financial and emotional needs of those who suffer great and often permanent harm."

The patient safety movement in the United States gained momentum with the seminal Institute of Medicine Report, *To Err is Human*.[14] The message from this report was that humans make mistakes and, to make the health care world safer, the focus must be on solutions to improve the underlying conditions that lead competent professionals to make those mistakes. Although this is true, one important element in that model is missing: the injured patient. While focusing on the future in harm prevention, health care systems must not forget the present in addressing the needs of the injured patient. Nancy Berlinger,[15] Deputy Director of Religious Studies at the Hastings Center, makes this point: "If the response to error is 'everyone makes mistakes'... this response is about the person who made the mistake, not about the persons who may be harmed by the mistake, and it utterly fails to address the aftermath of harmful mistakes."

DISCLOSURE LINKED TO SYSTEMS IMPROVEMENTS

Marcus and colleagues[16] queried patients who suffered harm from health care and concluded that patients expressed 3 significant needs from their health care provider after an event. Patients reported a desire for a full disclosure of what happened, a sincere apology, and assurance that actions were being implemented to prevent a similar occurrence with another patient in the future. Another study by Mazor[17] found that 88% of patients wanted an apology from their physicians, and 99% wanted to know that something was being done to prevent a similar adverse event in the future. Boothman[18] reports the benefits of integrating the Risk Management and Patient Safety programs at the University of Michigan with evidence that disclosure invariably becomes a component of broad systems improvement and is closely linked to improving patient safety. A robust risk management program active in the open disclosure of adverse events will be closely linked to an active patient safety program.[19] Patients who have been harmed demand systems improvements to prevent future harm to other patients.

DISCLOSURE: THE INTEGRATED TEAM APPROACH

Our experience in Lexington confirms that transparency and honesty in relationships with patients create opportunities for learning that lead to systems improvements in health care organizations. In the VHA, there are 3 categories of disclosure: clinical disclosure, institutional disclosure, and large-scale disclosure. The category of disclosure varies with the entity communicating the message, the reason for communicating the message, and the number of patients involved. Disclosures can be on a continuum as more information is learned about the adverse event.

Clinical disclosure exists within the framework of the provider-patient treatment relationship. It is information communicated by the treatment team, in the routine course of health care, for the purpose of providing relevant medical information to patients.[b] Institutional disclosure exists within the framework of the institution-veteran relationship, which is fundamental to the social contract the US Government has with the public to provide appropriate health care to veterans in exchange for service to their country. Serious harm or death from adverse events triggers the duty to conduct an institutional-level disclosure. Leaders with authority to speak on behalf of the organization formally accept responsibility for the patient harm, for the purpose of ameliorating the harm and improving the quality of health care in the institution. Large-scale disclosure exists in the context of a public health threat triggered by an adverse event that injures more than 3 patients. Communication of adverse event information is managed at the national level of the organization by coordinating with local medical centers to ensure rapid dissemination of information and remedial measures across the VHA (**Fig. 1**).

To honor our commitment to open disclosure and the legacy of the Lexington Model, we began to develop standardized disclosure practices and implement an integrated Risk Management and Patient Safety program in the Lexington VAMC in 2009. Our program was premised on the assumption that open disclosure is the natural derivative of our robust approach to ethics-based risk management and systems-based patient safety improvement. From November 2009 to August 2011 we conducted institutional disclosures with 20 patients or their personal representatives at the Lexington VAMC. Seventeen of those cases underwent a rigorous root cause analysis resulting in a multitude of systems improvements in the structure and processes of care.

When an incident occurs, it is reported into our electronic patient incident reporting system (ePIR).[c] A report can be entered in a few minutes with a simple click of an ePIR icon present on the desktop of all computers in the medical center. ePIR safety report categories are linked to the National Center for Patient Safety database.[20] Each report is reviewed and processed by the Patient Safety Manager (PSM) who communicates with the Chief of Performance Improvement (CPI) and the Risk Manager (RM). Should any member of our PSM/RM/CPI safety-risk team receive a report of an incident via informal means such as an e-mail, phone call, or face-to-face conversation, we ask the reporter to enter a report into ePIR. Our ePIR database serves as a final common pathway for incident reporting, creating a composite of all reported events, which allows our office to track events and assess for incidence and trends that may trigger a health care failure mode and effect analysis. All ePIR reports are summarized daily with senior leadership in a morning report as the first order of business.

---

[b] Clinical disclosure is indicated for adverse events that are expect to have a clinical effect on the patient that is perceptible to either the patient or the health care team; necessitate a change in the patient's care; have a known risk of serious future health consequences, even if the likelihood of that risk is extremely small; or require the provision of a treatment or procedure without the patient's consent.

[c] ePIR (developed for VAMCs by B.R. Smith, Jesse Brown VA Medical Center, Chicago, IL). Currently ePIR is used in more than 50 VAMCs nationwide.

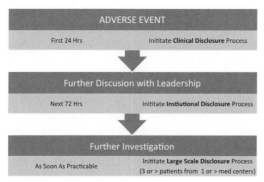

Fig. 1. Disclosure categories in the VHA.

When a report of an incident involves patient injury, our first concern is for the safety and well-being of our patient, and our second concern is to learn why it happened and how we can prevent it from happening again. Our team reviews the incident report and then activates pathways that may lead to disclosure, root cause analysis, or peer review (**Fig. 2**).

Disclosure and review can be a continuum of responses to an adverse event. The first step of the review is to check the veracity of the report and gather facts about the surrounding circumstances. The PSM requests the nurse manager or responsible physician to complete the report to document the clinical care of the patient and mitigation plans, if any had been implemented. After further initial investigation, the reporter or supervisor is invited to the Patient Safety Committee to discuss the case, where a recommendation is made to charter a root cause analysis or to embark on a rapid process improvement (RPI) action. RPIs are small process action teams that

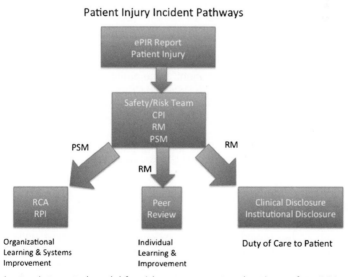

Fig. 2. Lexington integrated model for risk management and patient safety. RCA, root cause analysis; RPI, rapid process improvement.

conduct an intensive investigation and make recommendations to leadership for a mitigation plan in 1 or 2 meetings within 24 to 48 hours.

CLINICAL DISCLOSURE

The RM contacts the clinical team to inquire about the status of the patient and make an inquiry about whether a clinical disclosure had been done by the clinical team responsible for the patient. Clinical disclosures are an informal process for informing patients or their personal representatives of harmful adverse events related to the patient's care. Clinical disclosure is considered a normal activity in the course of medical practice in patient care and should be done within 24 hours of the incident, if possible. The VHA policy on adverse event disclosure requires a clinical disclosure to be documented in the patient's electronic medical record. Memorializing the clinical disclosure in a progress note is consistent with the VHA philosophy that clinical disclosure is like any other routine part of care and so should follow standard medical record documentation procedures.

INSTITUTIONAL DISCLOSURE

The RM convenes the medical center senior leadership who form the permanent Disclosure Team, the VHA staff attorney for the Regional Counsel Office, and any other necessary health care professionals, to discuss the appropriateness of an institutional disclosure. The Disclosure Team outlines the relevant information and identifies who should convey it to the patient. Institutional disclosures are a formal process of acknowledgment from the organization to patients or their personal representatives regarding harmful adverse events related to the patient's care. If the decision is to proceed, the RM office schedules an initial institutional disclosure meeting to be done within 72 hours of the incident, if possible. In most circumstances, it is difficult to ascertain the underlying cause of the incident without conducting further investigations. For this reason, institutional disclosure frequently requires a series of Institutional Disclosure Conferences (IDCs) or other personal contacts between the Disclosure Team and the patient to address the ongoing needs of the patient and family and to report the results of the investigation after it is completed (**Fig. 3**).

The IDC is conducted by the Chief of Staff, or designee, CPI, RM, and subject matter experts, such as the involved providers. Family members or friends may also attend at the discretion of the patient. If the patient chooses to have an attorney present, the VHA staff attorney for the Regional Counsel will also join the meeting. In the IDC meeting, the Disclosure Team divulges what happened to the extent that it is known, makes a sincere and empathic apology, and accepts responsibility on behalf of the medical center for what happened. The CPI provides a brief explanation of how the event will be prevented in the future or informs the patient that an investigation will be conducted for the purpose of preventing a future recurrence of a similar event.

The patient, family members, or friends affected by the adverse event are given an opportunity to express their feelings and thoughts about the experience and are encouraged to ask questions. Patient insight into the event commonly yields essential information about the underlying system issues. The RM advises patients of their rights to a second medical opinion, private legal representation, and to seek a remedy, if appropriate, by filing a federal tort and/or disability claim. After the IDC, the facility revenue manager is advised regarding the cancellation or hold on first-party and third-party billing for the relevant episode of care until the investigation has been

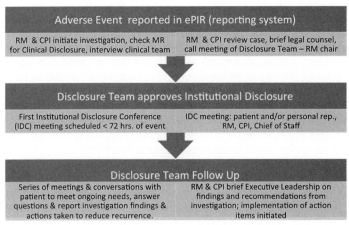

Fig. 3. Lexington model disclosure program from adverse event report to institutional disclosure.

completed. This process is described in the Lexington policy for disclosure of adverse events.[21]

After the initial IDC meeting, an investigation is launched and is usually completed in 4 to 6 weeks. The findings and recommendations from this process will be shared with the patient and family in a future meeting. In the meantime, interim measures are often taken to reduce the risk of recurrence and to mitigate further harm. The patient or personal representative is provided with contact information for members of the Disclosure Team and encouraged to call with any questions or concerns. All IDC conversations are documented in a special administrative institutional disclosure note that becomes a part of the patient's medical record. Key elements of the IDC meeting are described in **Fig. 4**.

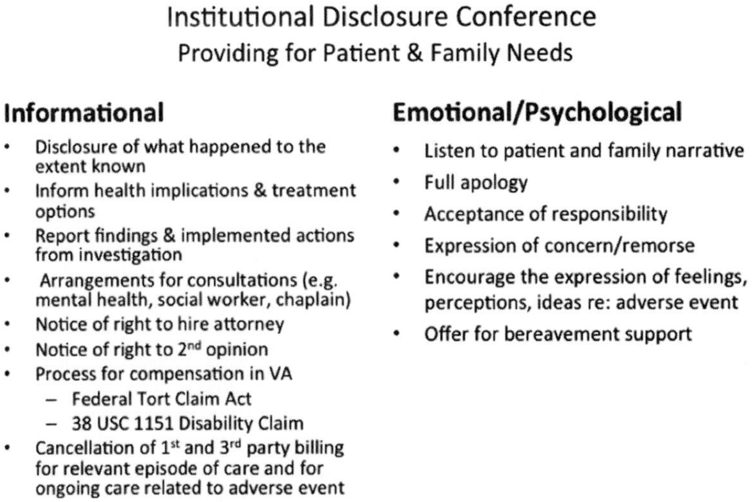

Institutional Disclosure Conference
Providing for Patient & Family Needs

Informational

- Disclosure of what happened to the extent known
- Inform health implications & treatment options
- Report findings & implemented actions from investigation
- Arrangements for consultations (e.g. mental health, social worker, chaplain)
- Notice of right to hire attorney
- Notice of right to 2nd opinion
- Process for compensation in VA
  - Federal Tort Claim Act
  - 38 USC 1151 Disability Claim
- Cancellation of 1st and 3rd party billing for relevant episode of care and for ongoing care related to adverse event

Emotional/Psychological

- Listen to patient and family narrative
- Full apology
- Acceptance of responsibility
- Expression of concern/remorse
- Encourage the expression of feelings, perceptions, ideas re: adverse event
- Offer for bereavement support

Fig. 4. IDC.

BARRIERS TO DISCLOSURE

Even with a robust integrated patient safety and risk management approach to disclosures, fear remains the major barrier for health care professionals to disclose adverse events. Institutional leaders and providers report fear of defending against a legal claim that is time consuming, embarrassing, and personally humiliating as a disincentive for disclosing information to a patient that might be used against the institution or provider.[d,22,23] A particular concern for providers is the possibility that a settled claim or a plaintiff jury award could result in the physician being reported to the National Practitioner Data Bank (NPDB). Physicians fear the NPDB report because professional reputation is so critical to successful medical practice.[e,24,25]

John Banja,[26] an ethicist from Emory University, asserts that rationalization and avoidance are psychological defenses to reduce distress and preserve self-esteem in the face of adverse events. Common rationalizations for not disclosing include that it will do more harm than good and that what really happened will never be known. Banja[26] argues that medical narcissism blocks disclosure because it emphasizes emotional distance from the patient, the need for clinician control, and an excessive focus on disease and treatment with inattention to the person. As a result, many physicians lack empathic communication skills because they have a strong need to control patients' thoughts, feelings, and decisions. Listening is a critical part of disclosure that is often not well developed among physicians. Banja[26] believes that physicians need training in empathic communication, and that senior administrators need training in managing disclosure from a patient-centered perspective.[26] The author (EJD), a practicing cardiovascular surgeon for 20 years, corroborates Banja's[26] observations from anecdotal experience and observations of colleagues in the hospital setting.

So, are the fears of health care professionals grounded in reality or are these myths perpetuated over time and passed from one generation to the next? Fear of a lawsuit is on the minds of clinicians when making medical decisions, but how much impact does it have? A survey of 2637 physicians and surgeons in the United States concluded that medical liability fears had a minimal impact on the physicians' willingness to disclose an error to the patient.[22] Results from the same study were reviewed to see what conditions did affect error disclosure and it was determined that attitudes about error disclosure were dominated by the culture of the physicians more than the fear of being sued.[22] In addition, malpractice premiums and awards consume a small percentage of the health economy. Less than 1% of patients who have suffered adverse events from substandard care (ie, negligent harm) have a successful claim against the provider. Most malpractice claims do not involve provider negligence, and most patients who were victims of negligent care never file a tort claim.[27]

---

[d] Wide variation existed regarding what information respondents would disclose. Of the respondents, 56% chose statements that mentioned the adverse event but not the error, whereas 42% would explicitly state that an error occurred. Some physicians disclosed little information: 19% would not volunteer any information about the error's cause, and 63% would not provide specific information about preventing future errors. Disclosure was affected by the nature of the error and physician specialty. Of the respondents, 51% who received the more apparent errors explicitly mentioned the error, compared with 32% who received the less apparent errors (P<.001); 58% of medical specialists explicitly mentioned the error, compared with 19% of surgical specialists (P<.001). Respondents disclosed more information if they had positive disclosure attitudes, thought they were responsible for the error, had prior positive disclosure experiences, and were Canadian.

[e] Although participants knew they should report errors associated with serious adverse events, both physicians and nurses agreed that reporting was intended to change practice and policy to promote patient safety.

THE COOPERATION CLAUSE OF EMPLOYMENT AND INSURANCE CONTRACTS

A common concern among physicians who do not have protection under the Federal Tort Claim Act is the risk of losing malpractice insurance coverage if an adverse event is disclosed to a patient.[f,28] The fear comes from the possible interpretation that a disclosure is an admission of wrongdoing that could interfere with the insurer's defense against the plaintiff's claim. Proponents of the deny-and-defend paradigm may view full disclosure of an adverse event as a violation of the insured party's (MD) obligation to cooperate with the insurer and not collude with the injured party. Any contractual provision prohibiting truthful communications with patients about relevant health care issues is clearly against public policy and would be difficult to enforce.[9,29] In contrast, it is unambiguous that collusion with an insurer to deceive patients is unlawful. When faced with a cooperation clause in an insurance policy, a physician could make a strong argument for a moral obligation to disclose an adverse event.

An employer, such as the VHA, does have the right to require employee providers to cooperate with institutional disclosure policies. Employer rights are qualified by the provider's duty to the patient and ability to practice medicine within the scope of his authority. An employer does not have the right to force or coerce a provider to refrain from a clinical disclosure against the weight of the provider's independent medical judgment about the patient's best interests. The provider's judgment would be measured against the norms established by the profession.

The plausibility of a cooperation clause becoming a deterrent to open disclosure is diminished when compared with the impact of a perceived cover-up. Discovery of a concealed adverse event would likely be far more costly to an insurance company or institution in terms of reputational harm and reduced ability to prevail in court than the settlement of a claim resulting from open and honest disclosure done in a timely fashion.

Behavioral change that embraces adverse event disclosure might only be achievable on a comprehensive organizational level. Such organizational change would be predicated on creating a supportive environment for physicians when their patients sustain adverse events and offering them training in empathic communication skills with strategies for effective disclosure experiences for patients and families. Our Disclosure Team in Lexington supports physicians and nurses whose patients have experienced adverse events, including our presence in clinical disclosure meetings when requested. These meetings can be the most difficult conversations a clinician will ever experience in practice.

REMOVING BARRIERS

A proactive method to address the fear of adverse event disclosure that permeates most health care institutions is to break the code of silence by standardizing the

---

[f] Government liability for a tort is limited by the sovereign immunity doctrine. To preserve the Government's ability to function, which is for the greater good of the public writ large, citizens are prohibited from suing the Government and its employees. An exception to the doctrine applies in cases in which the Government has explicitly or implicitly consented to be sued. The Federal Tort Claim Act (FTCA) explicitly authorizes tort claims, based on state law, to be brought against the Government for tortious conduct against private citizens. This exception allows patients to bring limited medical negligence claims against the Government for care rendered by the VA as health care provider, but shields all employees from being sued if they are acting within the scope of their employment.

[g] In *Ritter*, the Supreme Court ruled that any insurance policy, "the tendency of which is to endanger the public interests or injuriously affect the public good, or which is subversive of sound morality, ought never to receive the sanction of a court of justice or be made the foundation of its judgment."

policies, procedures, and practice of disclosures and raising the expectation for compliance. The early inspirational work of Kraman and Hamm informed national VHA policy in the open disclosure of adverse events culminating in a national directive issued in January 2008,[30] but efforts to operationalize the policy have been inconsistent in facilities across the VHA.

Disclosure practice in Lexington continued in an informal manner with less notoriety in the aftermath of the retirement of Kraman (2003) and Hamm (2009) from the Lexington VAMC. The authors have been managing the Lexington Open Disclosure Program since November 2009. In that 21-month period, 20 institutional disclosures have been conducted. Most of these disclosure cases highlighted significant systems vulnerabilities requiring root cause analysis teams in 17 of the 20 cases, which led to a multitude of improvements in patient safety. However, only 6 clinical disclosures could be documented in the medical records of these patients. Four tort claims were filed and all settled for amounts ranging from $2500 (minor wrong patient procedure) to $750,000 (serious injury or death), respectively. One patient filed a federal disability claim. Of the 17 surviving patients, all continue to seek their health care needs at the Lexington VAMC, and many of these patients remain in contact with our office and call if they need help with issues related to accessing services in the medical center.

During that same time period, medical center policies on adverse event disclosure, quality improvement, patient safety, and ethics-based risk management were drafted and implemented. The disclosure practice was formalized, monitored for performance improvement opportunities, and refined based on stakeholder feedback. In June of 2011, education for staff on adverse event policy and procedure was initiated for all employees starting with critical services, defined by tort claim data. The goal of behavioral change that supports the standardization of disclosure of adverse events to patients and their families as part of the routine practice of medicine has moved to a national level.

The authors have developed an Open Disclosure Training Program (ODTP). The program is funded by a Systems Improvement Capability Grant[h,31] from the VHA to develop a standardized, replicable method for teaching clinicians and administrators how to deliver a disclosure message explaining adverse events or medical mistakes to patients and families. The program uses an integrated structure of classroom instruction with film vignettes depicting health care provider interactions with patients and other providers and disclosure simulations with actors.

The target audience for the program includes physicians, nurses, allied health personnel, health profession students, VHA attorneys, and health administrators. The purpose of this training program is to establish a consistent, high-quality disclosure experience for patients and families in the VHA. We plan to model disclosure practice for adverse events from medical care including events caused by mistakes in the delivery of care. This training program will be offered to the Lexington VAMC and be exportable to other health care institutions. Improvements in patient outcomes of care and provider job satisfaction will be achieved through the implementation of the ODTP. By eliminating waste, improving underlying systems, increasing teamwork coordination, and honoring our ethical duty to disclose, we will enhance the delivery of ethics-based, patient-centered health care.

---

[h] The Lexington VAMC is the recipient of a 3-year Systems Improvement Capability Grant funded by the VHA from 2010 to 2012. A major focus of the grant is on the development of an ODTP based on experiential learning that will culminate in a 2-day workshop of didactics, facilitated interactive dialogue, training films produced by the ODTP team of clinical scenarios to stimulate dialogue on various aspects of disclosure, and simulations of disclosure by attendees with professional actors facilitated by faculty.

SUMMARY

Inspired by the pioneering work of the original Lexington Model, and compelled by our ethical, professional, and legal duties to disclose, this article outlines an enhanced integrated team approach to the Open Disclosure Program in Lexington. From its inception, the ultimate goal of this program was to seek and achieve just outcomes for patients and providers, which remains the goal of our program today. The value of an integrated approach to patient-centered risk management and patient safety is shown by our success in meeting patient and organizational expectations to improve care after an adverse event. Further empirical study is needed to validate our initial observations of the positive organizational impact from standardization of our integrated disclosure practices.

We conclude from our experience thus far that, while focusing on future harm prevention, the present needs of the injured patient must not be neglected. A just outcome requires provider support from the health care institution when an adverse event occurs, improvement of the underlying conditions to enhance the safety of care, an opportunity of forgiveness from the patient for harm caused by the adverse event, and fair compensation. By rejecting the old paradigm of silence and secrecy

---

Disclosure to a surgical patient

WS, a 70-year-old man, underwent a low anterior resection for carcinoma of the sigmoid colon via open laparotomy. The procedure was complicated by pelvic bleeding, which was controlled surgically and required a 2-unit transfusion of packed red blood cells. The patient did well after surgery for the first 24 hours. On the first postoperative day, a plain film of the abdomen revealed what appeared to be a 4×4 sponge in the pelvis as reported by a radiologist. The surgeon reviewed the film and concurred with this finding. He informed the RM and planned a meeting with the patient and his family as soon as it could be arranged.

The surgeon and RM met with the patient and family at the bedside on the medical-surgical unit. He sat down on a chair at the bedside and calmly explained the radiographic finding. He advised WS to undergo reoperation for removal of the sponge because of the long-term risk of health consequences for leaving a sponge in the abdominal cavity, such as abdominal abscess and bowel obstruction. He apologized and took responsibility for what happened and mentioned that a team was being organized to investigate this case. The patient and his wife were alarmed and questioned how a sponge could be left in the abdomen but accepted the surgeon's recommendation. Later that afternoon, WS underwent an exploratory laparotomy, and the sponge was removed. He did well after surgery and was discharged home in 5 days.

Senior leadership met with the Disclosure Team 24 hours after the event and granted approval to proceed with institutional disclosure, which was initiated 24 hours later. Leadership also approved the cancellation of first-party and third-party billing for services rendered during the current hospitalization. The Institutional disclosure conference meeting was conducted by the Associate Chief of Staff and the Risk Manager with WS, his wife, and their daughter. On behalf of the medical center, the Disclosure Team explained what happened and offered a full apology with acceptance of responsibility. They affirmed the patient's right to a second medical opinion and to hire an attorney. They advised the patient of his right to pursue a legal remedy if he wished via federal tort claim and/or disability claim and would provide the forms for each. The patient was informed that all first-party and third-party billing for services during his present hospitalization were canceled.

WS continued to seek his health care from the same medical center with which his primary care provider had an affiliation. He called the RM with a question about his medical bill and also asked for her help to obtain an appointment in the Ophthalmology Clinic. In a follow-up meeting 6 weeks later, the Disclosure Team reported the findings and recommendations from the investigative team. Several measures were being implemented to reduce the likelihood of a retained surgical sponge in another patient in the future.

following an adverse event and making open disclosure of adverse events to patients and their families a part of the routine practice of medicine, real transparency can be promoted. Transparency is the foundation for trust between patient and provider and is also necessary for organizational learning, which is the basis for improving the safety of health care organizations for the patients they serve.

REFERENCES

1. VHA Directive 2008-002. Disclosure of adverse events to patients. (January 18, 2008). Available at: http://www.va.gov/vhapublications/ViewPublication.asp?pub_ID=1637. Accessed July 27, 2011.
2. Griffin FD. The impact of transparency on patient safety and liability. Bull Am Coll Surg 2008;93(3):19–23.
3. Kraman S, Hamm G. Risk management: extreme honesty may be the best policy. Ann Intern Med 1999;131(12):963–7.
4. Hamm G, Kraman S. New standards, new dilemmas – reflections on managing medical mistakes. Bioethics Forum 2001;17(2):19–25.
5. Beauchamp T, Childress J. Principles of biomedical ethics. New York: Oxford University Press; 2001.
6. American College of Physicians. Must you disclose mistakes made by other physicians? Case study by ACP Ethics and Human Rights Committee and Professionalism. 2003. Available at: http://www.acponline.org/journals/news/nov03/mistakes.htm. Accessed July 15, 2011.
7. Johnstone MJ, Kanitsaki O. The ethics and practical importance of defining, distinguishing and disclosing nursing errors: a discussion paper. Int J Nurs Stud 2006;43:367–76.
8. Council on Ethical and Judicial Affairs. Code of medical ethics: current opinions with annotations. 2002-3 edition. Chicago: AMA Press; 2002. p. 217–8.
9. Woods M. Healing words – the power of apology in medicine. Oak Park (IL): Doctors in Touch; 2004. p. 16.
10. Sage W, Zivin J, Chase N. Bridging the relational-regulatory gap. Vanderbilt Legal Review 2006;59:1263.
11. Joint Commission. Comprehensive Accreditation Manual for Hospitals. 2011.
12. Banja J. Medical errors and medical narcissism. Sudbury (MD): Jones and Bartlett; 2005.
13. Levine C. Life but no limb: the aftermath of medical error. Health Aff (Millwood) 2002;21(4):237–41.
14. Kohn L, Corrigan J, Donaldson M. To err is human: building a safer healthcare system. Washington, DC: Institute of Medicine, National Academy Press; 2000.
15. Berlinger N. After harm – medical error and the ethics of forgiveness. Baltimore (MD): Johns Hopkins University Press; 2005.
16. Marcus L, Dorn B, McNulty E. Renegotiating health care: resolving conflict to build collaboration. 2nd edition. San Francisco (CA): Jossey-Bass; 2011.
17. Mazor K. The health plan members' views about disclosure of medical errors. Ann Intern Med 2004;140(6):409–18.
18. Boothman R. Medical justice: making the system work better for patients and doctors. Testimony before the United States Senate Committee on Health, Education, Labor and Pensions, June 22, 2006. Available at: http://help.senate.gov/imo/media/doc/boothman.pdf. Accessed December 12, 2011.
19. Boothman R. Integrating risk management activities into a patient safety program. Clin Obstet Gynecol 2010;53:576–85.

20. VA National Center for Patient Safety. Ann Arbor (MI). Available at: www. patientsafety.gov. Accessed July 15, 2011.
21. Lexington VA Medical Center. Available at: http://vaww.lexington.med.va.gov/ docs/memo.aspx. Accessed August 3, 2011.
22. Gallagher TH, Waterman AD, Garbutt JM, et al. US and Canadian physicians' attitudes and experiences regarding disclosing errors to patients. Arch Intern Med 2006;166(15):1605–11.
23. Gallagher TH, Garbutt JM, Waterman AD, et al. Choosing your words carefully: how physicians would disclose harmful medical errors to patients. Arch Intern Med 2006;166(15):1585–93.
24. Jeffe DB, Dunagan WC, Garbutt J, et al. Using focus groups to understand physicians' and nurses' perspectives on error reporting in hospitals. Jt Comm J Qual Saf 2004;30(9):471–9.
25. Kaldjian LC, Jones EW, Rosenthal GE. Facilitating and impeding factors for physicians' error disclosure: a structured literature review. Jt Comm J Qual Patient Saf 2006;32(4):188–98.
26. Banja J. Medical Errors and Medical Narcissism. Sudbury (MA): Jones and Bartlett Publishers; 2005.
27. Studdert D, Mello M, Brennan T. Medical malpractice. N Engl J Med 2004;350(3): 283–92 All2.
28. See Recinto v U.S. Department of Veterans Affairs, N.D.Cal. 4-28-2011 (2011).
29. Ritter v Mutual Live Ins. Co. (Supreme Court 1898), quoted in Dobbyn JF, 1996. p. 107.
30. Veterans Health Administration. Available at: http://www1.va.gov/vhapublications/ ViewPublication.asp?pub_ID=1637. Accessed July 15, 2011.
31. Dunn E, Eaves-Leanos, McKinney K, et al. Re-engineering organizational learning to optimize veteran-centered care. Systems Improvement Capability Grant submission in August 2009 accessed on the Veterans Health Administration Systems Redesign. Available at: https://srd.vssc.med.va.gov/Committee/si/ ImprovementGrant/Pages/default-old.aspx. Accessed December 12, 2011.

Index

Note: Page numbers of article titles are in **boldface** type.

A

Accreditation Council for Graduate Medical Education (ACGME)
  described, 117
  regulations of
    current system, 118
      alternatives to, 118–119
  in residency training
    evaluation of
      Libby Zion and, 118
Accreditation Council for Graduate Medical Education (ACGME) reforms
  history and legacy of, **117–123**
  limited observation on, 119
  regulations of
    types of, 119
ACGME. *See* Accreditation Council for Graduate Medical Education (ACGME)
Adverse events
  open disclosure of, **163–177**
    barriers to, 172
      removal of, 173–174
    clinical disclosure, 168, 170
    cooperation clause of employment and insurance contracts, 173
    described, 163–164
    ethical obligation for, 164–165
    institutional disclosure, 170–171
    integrated team approach to, 167–170
    as legal and regulatory mandate, 166
    patient safety as factor in, 166–167
    as professional duty, 165–166
    reasons for, 164
    to surgical patient, 175
    systems improvement as factor in, 167
  surgeons' reactions to, **153–161**
    difficulty with error disclosure, 158–159
    example of, 153–155
    framework for understanding, 155
    future directions related to, 159
    learning from, 157–158
    operating after complication, 157
    phases of, 155–156
    placing framework into context, 156–159
  surgery-related, **89–100**

Surg Clin N Am 92 (2012) 179–188
doi:10.1016/S0039-6109(12)00009-6
0039-6109/12/$ – see front matter © 2012 Elsevier Inc. All rights reserved.

surgical.theclinics.com

Adverse (*continued*)
    examples of, 89–90, 98–99
    latent factors and, 90–91
    multiple causes analysis in, 95–97
    person approach to
        consequences of, 97
    RCA investigations of
        making sense of, **101–115**. *See also* Root cause analysis (RCA), of
            surgery-related adverse events
    RCA methods in, 92–94
    root causes of, 90–91
    secrecy, malpractice, and error in, 97
    theories of error in, 91–92
Agency for Healthcare Researchers and Quality (AHRQ)
    in measuring quality in surgery, 57–59
AHRQ. *See* Agency for Healthcare Researchers and Quality (AHRQ)
Automated data collection
    patient safety and, 84

    B

Bar code technology, 82–83
Behavioral markers systems, 38–39
Bias
    unconscious
        in surgical safety and outcomes, **137–151**. *See also* Unconscious bias

    C

Catheter-associated urinary tract infection (CAUTI), 71–73
Catheter-related bloodstream infection (CRBSI), 66–68
    costs related to, 67
    defined, 66
    diagnosis of, 66
    epidemiology of, 67
    mechanisms of, 67
    microbiology of, 67
    prevention of, 68
    quality improvement for patients with, 68
    risk factors for, 67
    treatment of, 67
CAUTI. *See* Catheter-associated urinary tract infection (CAUTI)
Clinical disclosure
    of adverse events, 168, 170
Clinical microsystems, **7–11**
    described, 7–9
    leadership in
        patient safety and, 9
    patient safety and, 9
    surgical microsystems
        designing safe
            recommendations and principles for, 10–11

Communication
  in NOTSS project, 44–45
  in OR, 24–27
  in surgery
    improving, 56
Comprehensive unit-based safety program (CUSP)
  in surgery, **51–63**
    measuring quality, 57–61
      AHRQ in, 57–59
      NSQIP in, 60–61
      PSIs in, 58
      SCIP in, 59–60
      standardization of patient safety terminology, 57
    never events, 52
    protocols and culture changes to prevent error, 54–56
    science for, 51–52
    wrong-site/wrong-patient surgery, 52–53
Computerized physician order entry (CPOE), 80
Contract(s)
  employment and insurance
    cooperation clause of
      in open disclosure of adverse events, 173
CPOE. *See* Computerized physician order entry (CPOE)
CRBSI. *See* Catheter-related bloodstream infection (CRBSI)
CUSP. *See* Comprehensive unit-based safety program (CUSP)

D

Data collection
  automated
    patient safety and, 84
Disclosure
  clinical, 168, 170
  error, 158–159
  institutional, 170–171
  open
    of adverse events, **163–177**. *See also* Adverse events, open disclosure of

E

EHRs. *See* Electronic health records (EHRs)
Electronic health records (EHRs)
  described, 79
  for surgical care
    implementation of, 80–82
Employment contracts
  cooperation clause of
    in open disclosure of adverse events, 173
Error disclosure
  of surgical adverse event
    difficulty of, 158–159

Ethics
  as factor in disclosure related to adverse events, 164–165

F

Fall
  as surgeon's reaction to adverse event, 155–156
Fatigue
  in NOTSS project, 47
Fishbone diagram
  in RCA, 92
5 whys
  in RCA, 92–94

H

HACs. *See* Hospital-acquired conditions (HACs)
HAIs. *See* Hospital-acquired infections (HAIs)
Health information technology
  bar code technology, 82–83
  EHR implementation in, 80–82
Health Information Technology for Economic and Clinical Health (HITECH) Act, 79
  described, 79–80
High-performance teams
  in operating room, **15–19**. *See also* Operating room (OR), high-performance teams in
High reliability organizations (HROs), **1–7**
  brittleness of, 2
  described, 1–2
  law of stretched systems, 2
  principles of, 3–5
    commitment to resilience, 2, 4
    deference to expertise, 4–5
    preoccupation with failure, 3
    reluctance to simplify, 3
    sensitivity to operations, 3–4
  resilience of, 2, 4
  teamwork and, 6–7
HITECH. *See* Health Information Technology for Economic and Clinical Health (HITECH) Act
Hospital-acquired conditions (HACs). *See also* Hospital-acquired infections (HAIs)
  described, 65
Hospital-acquired infections (HAIs), **65–77**. *See also specific types, e.g.,* Catheter-related bloodstream infection (CRBSI)
  CAUTI, 71–73
  costs related to, 65
  CRBSI, 66–68
  incidence of, 65–66
  mortality data, 65–66
  SSI, 70–71
  VAP, 68–69
HROs. *See* High reliability organizations (HROs)

Human factors
in operating room safety, **21–35**. *See also* Operating room (OR)

I

Information technologies. *See also specific types, e.g.,* Health information technology
patient safety and, **79–87**
automated data collection, 84
bar code technology, 82–83
EHR implementation, 80–82
intraoperative monitoring, 83–84
RFID, 82–83
RSIs, 82–83
Institutional disclosure
of adverse events, 170–171
Insurance contracts
cooperation clause of
in open disclosure of adverse events, 173
Intraoperative monitoring
patient safety and, 83–84

K

Kick
as surgeon's reaction to adverse event, 155

L

Leadership
in NOTSS project, 45–46
Legal issues
in open disclosure of adverse events, 166
Long-term impact
as surgeon's reaction to adverse event, 156

M

Malpractice
surgical error and, 97
Medical error
person approach to
consequences of, 97
Microsystem(s)
clinical, **7–11**. *See also* Clinical microsystems
Multiple causes analysis
of adverse events, 95–97

N

National Surgical Quality Improvement Program (NSQIP)
in measuring quality in surgery, 60–61

Never events
    in surgery, 52
Non-technical skills
    of surgeons, **37–50**. *See also* Surgeon(s), non-technical skills of
NOTECHS, 38–39
NOTSS project, 39–47
    categories of, 42–47
    decision making in, 43–44
    described, 39–40
    development of, 39
    fatigue in, 47
    leadership in, 45–46
    SA in, 40–43
    stress in, 46–47
    surgical checklist in, 46
    teamwork and communication in, 44–45
NSQIP. *See* National Surgical Quality Improvement Program (NSQIP)

O

ODTP. *See* Open Disclosure Training Program (ODTP)
Open disclosure
    of adverse events, **163–177**. *See also* Adverse events, open disclosure of
Open Disclosure Training Program (ODTP), 174
Operating room (OR)
    environment of, 22–24
    high-performance teams in
        building of, **15–19**
        development of, 16
        learning from those that do it well, 15–16
        practical interventions for, 17–18
        return on investment, 18–19
    improving leadership engagement in, 31
    layout of, 22–23
    noise in, 23–24
    organizational influences in, 30–32
    safety of
        described, 21–22
        human factors and, **21–35**
    surgeon's role in, 31–32
    task and workload factors in, 29–30
    teamwork and communication in, 24–27
        cumulative experience, familiarity, and stability of, 25–26
        preoperative briefings, 26–27
    tools and technology in, 27–29
Operative judgment
    slowing-down moments of
        expertise and, 128–131
        manifestations of, 128–130
        teaching of, **125–135**
            implications of, 132–133

proactively planned slowing-down moments, 132–133
situationally responsive slowing-down moments, 133
surgeon educator in, 131–132
theoretical framework of, 126–128
attention and effort in, 126–127
SA in, 127–128
types of
categorization of, 130–131
OR. *See* Operating room (OR)
OSATS, 40
OTAS, 38

P

Patient safety. *See also* Safety
clinical microsystems and, 9
as factor in open disclosure of adverse events, 166–167
information technologies and, **79–87**. *See also specific technologies and* Information
technologies, patient safety and
intraoperative monitoring and, 83–84
Patient safety indicators (PSIs)
in surgery, 58
Pneumonia
ventilator-associated, 68–69
PSIs. *See* Patient safety indicators (PSIs)

R

Radiofrequency identification (RFID)
in reducing RSIs in patient safety, 82–83
RCA. *See* Root cause analysis (RCA)
Recovery
as surgeon's reaction to adverse event, 156
Residency training
ACGME oversight of
evaluation of
Libby Zion and, 118
in surgery
oversights in, **117–123**
Libby Zion, 118
safety culture and handoffs, 120
unanswered questions and unintended consequences, 119–120
work hours and education, 120–122
Retained surgical items (RSIs)
reducing of
in patient safety, 82–83
RFID. *See* Radiofrequency identification (RFID)
Root cause analysis (RCA)
of surgery-related adverse events, 92–94, **101–115**
in altering improvement capability of surgical centers, 105–109
fishbone diagram in, 92–94

Root (*continued*)
    5 whys in, 92–94
    focus on
       health care effects of, 112
    historical background of, 101–104
    indications for, 99
    limitations of
       responding to, 109–112
    in measuring safety, 105
    usefulness of, 97
RSIs. *See* Retained surgical items (RSIs)

S

SA. *See* Situation awareness (SA)
Safety
    in health care
       transparency and, **163–177**. *See also* Adverse events, open disclosure of
    in surgery
       assessment of, 55–56
       barriers to improved, 54–55
       improving teamwork and communication, 56
       standardization of terminology related to, 57
       unconscious bias' role in, **137–151**. *See also* Unconscious bias
    in surgical residency training
       oversights in, 120
SCIP. *See* Surgical Care Improvement Project (SCIP)
Secrecy
    in surgical error, 97
Situation awareness (SA)
    in NOTSS project, 40–43
    in teaching slowing-down moments of operative judgment, 127–128
SSI. *See* Surgical site infection (SSI)
Stress
    in NOTSS project, 46–47
Stretched systems
    law of, 2
Surgeon(s)
    non-technical skills of, **37–50**
       behavioral markers systems, 38–39
       described, 37–38
    role in OR, 31–32
    when bad things happen to, **153–161**. *See also* Adverse events
Surgery
    adverse events related to, **89–100**. *See also* Adverse events
    CUSP in, **51–63**. *See also* Comprehensive unit-based safety program (CUSP), in surgery
    error in, **89–100**. *See also* Adverse events
       person approach to
          consequences of, 97
       protocols and culture changes in prevention of, 54–56
    judgment during

teaching slowing-down moments of, **125–135**. *See also* Operative judgment, slowing-down moments of, teaching of

quality of

measuring of, 57–61. *See also* Comprehensive unit-based safety program (CUSP), in surgery, measuring quality

residency training in

oversights in, **117–123**. *See also* Residency training, in surgery

safety related to. *See* Patient safety; Safety; Surgical safety

Surgical care

adverse events in, **89–100**. *See also* Adverse events

EHR implementation for, 80–82

Surgical Care Improvement Project (SCIP)

in measuring quality in surgery, 59–60

Surgical centers

improvement capability of

RCA in altering, 105–109

Surgical checklist

in NOTSS project, 46

Surgical microsystems

designing safe

recommendations and principles for, 10–11

Surgical safety. *See also* Patient safety; Safety

unconscious bias' role in, **137–151**. *See also* Unconscious bias

Surgical site infection (SSI), 70–71

System improvement

as factor in open disclosure of adverse events, 167

T

Task and workload factors

in OR, 29–30

Teamwork

in NOTSS project, 44–45

in OR, 24–27

in surgery

improving, 56

Tools and technology

in OR, 27–29

Transparency

in health care

safety and, **163–177**. *See also* Adverse events, open disclosure of

U

Unconscious bias

effect on physician-patient encounter, 142

in experimental studies, 140–142

in medicine

described, 138–139

in naturalistic studies, 139–140

in surgical safety and outcomes, **137–151**

Unconscious (*continued*)
    reducing of, 142–144
Urinary tract infection (UTI)
    catheter-associated, 71–73
UTI. *See* Urinary tract infection (UTI)

V

VAP. *See* Ventilator-associated pneumonia (VAP)
Ventilator-associated pneumonia (VAP), 68–69

W

Wrong-site/wrong-patient surgery, 52–53

Z

Zion, Libby
    evaluation of ACGME oversight in residency training and, 118